The Microbiome Diet Plan

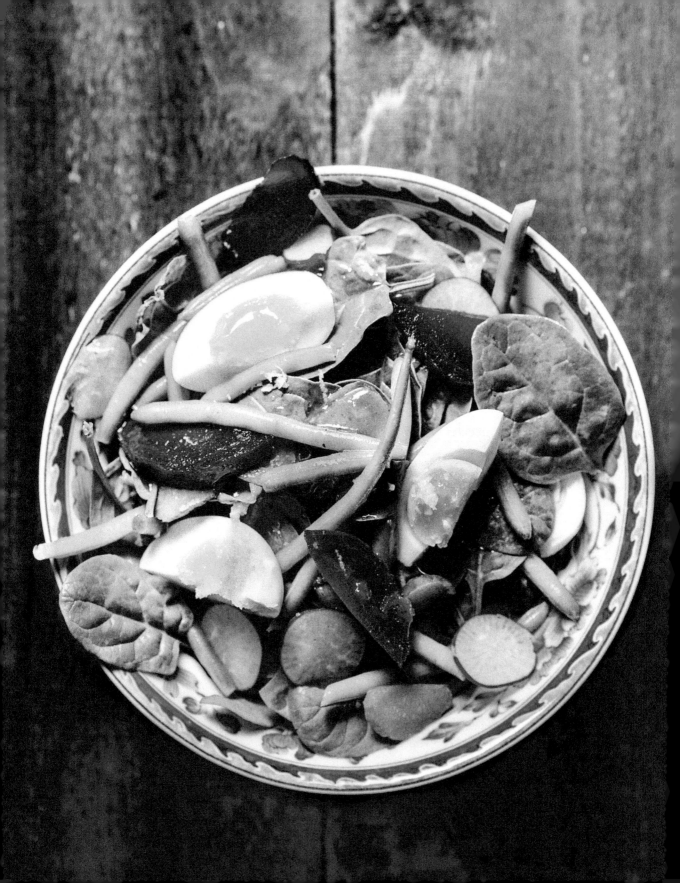

The Microbiome Diet Plan

SIX WEEKS to LOSE WEIGHT and IMPROVE YOUR GUT HEALTH

Danielle Capalino, MSPH, RD, CDN

ROCKRIDGE PRESS

For general information on our other products and services or to obtain technical support, please contact our Customer Care Department within the U.S. at (866) 744-2665, or outside the U.S. at (510) 253-0500.

Rockridge Press publishes its books in a variety of electronic and print formats. Some content that appears in print may not be available in electronic books, and vice versa.

Photography © Darren Muir/Stocksy, p.2; Eric van Lokven/StockFood, p6; Martí Sans/Stocksy, p.9; Marta Muñoz-Calero Calderon/Stocksy, p.10; Don Crossland/Stockfood, p.12; Rua Castilho/Stockfood, p.22; marekuliasz/Shutterstock, p.34; Nataša Mandić/Stocksy, p.36; Nadine Greeff/Stocksy, p.50; BONNINSTUDIO/Stocksy, p.65; Lumina/Stocksy, p.66; Charlotte Tolhurst/Stockfood, p.68; Ellie Baygulov/Stocksy, p.92; Theresa Raffetto/Stockfood, p.118; Shaun Cato-Symonds/Stockfood, p.142; Gareth Morgans/Stockfood, p.156; Rua Castilho/Stockfood, p.176; Gräfe & Unzer Verlag/Mona Binner Photographie/Stockfood, p.194; Spyros Bourboulis/Stockfood, p.208; Canan Czemmel/Stocksy, p.220; Eric Van Lokven/Stockfood, p.232.
Cover clockwise from top: HandmadePictures/Shutterstock; stockcreations/Shutterstock; ch_ch/Shutterstock; Lumina/Stocksy; The Picture Pantry/Stockfood.
Back cover from top: Shaun Cato-Symonds/Stockfood; Darren Muir/Stocksy; Photo of the author by Jami Saunders

ISBN: Print 978-1-62315-866-8 | eBook 978-1-62315-867-5

*To my mother, who willed this book
to happen with her voodoo power.*

What should I write about next?

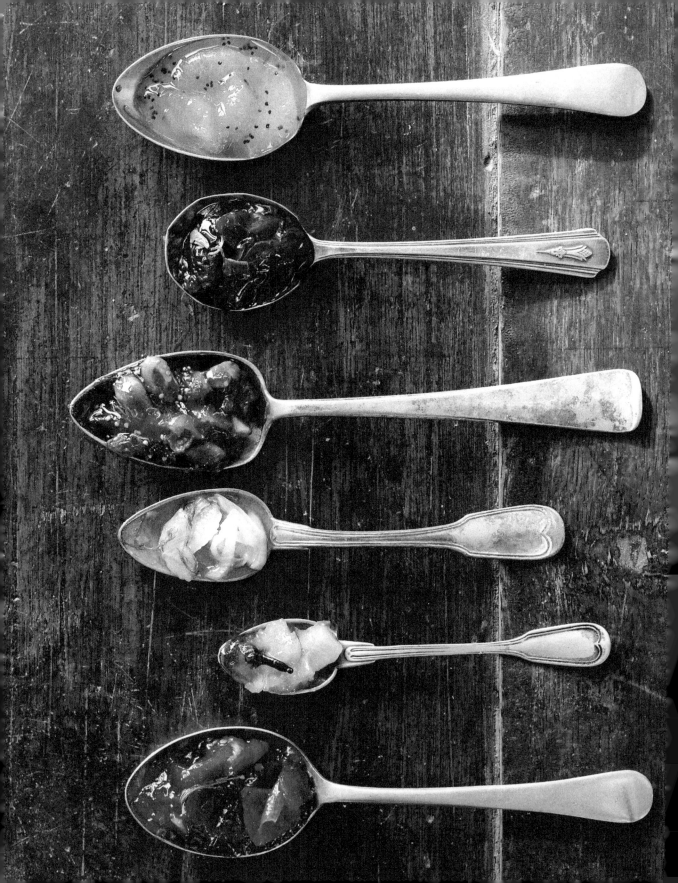

Contents

Introduction

Why should you care about microbes? One answer is sheer numbers—a statistic that many scientists have referenced is that bacteria outnumber human cells in the human body by a factor of ten to one. Though that has recently been called into question, by any measure we have an enormous amount of bacteria that live on our skin and in our guts, as well as in other parts of the body. This massive collection of microorganisms, largely thought of as bacteria (though it also includes viruses and fungi), is known as the microbiome. Over the past several years, research on the microbiome has exploded, linking a healthy microbiome to a healthy body weight and the absence of allergies and disease.

Sounds great, right? If we all had the perfect microbiome, we would be thin and healthy. If only it were that simple! The truth is we do not yet know what the perfect—or even normal—microbiome looks like, or if that even exists. But what we do know is that what we eat plays a tremendous role in shaping the community of organisms in our guts. We also know that there are changes that you can make today to improve the quality of your microbiome. Scientific studies examining how food influences the microbiome are still very new: I'm here to tell you what we know and what we don't know.

When I began to learn about the immense power of the microbiome, my life changed. It was 2009 and I had gone back to school to formally study nutrition. The world of the microbiome was brand-new—not yet in the headlines. My microbiology professor gave me a paper to read about the role of the microbiome in obesity, and that paper turned the entire premise of nutrition (that body weight is based on calories in and calories out) on its head. This was groundbreaking, and in that moment I knew my course of study in nutrition was going to focus on the role of the microbiome: the long-ignored vital component that influences our health and our weight.

With this evidence in hand, I launched a quest to learn everything I could about the power of bacteria in our guts and what it can do to help us get or stay healthy. I went on to continue my study of the gut microbiome in graduate school at Johns Hopkins Bloomberg School of Public Health and in my dietetic internship at Johns Hopkins. I studied with Dr. Gerard Mullin, a professor at Johns Hopkins and pioneer in digestive health and nutrition. I learned firsthand as I saw the impact of the microbiome on the gastrointestinal health of his patients. After graduating, I moved home to New York City to start a thriving private practice to help people attain

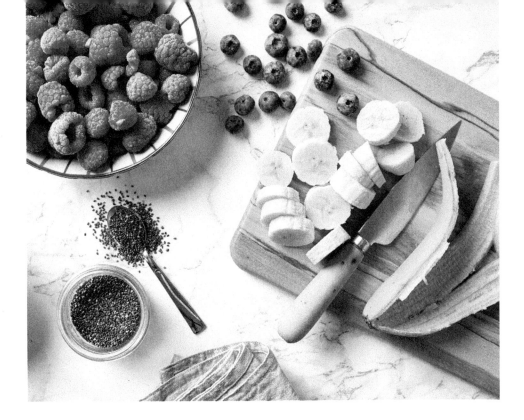

digestive health through diet. I wanted to be able to share the results of this promising scientific inquiry with people who were struggling and seeking help.

And that's where this book comes in. First, you're going to get the 411 on the microbiome and its role in health and disease. I will explain the science linking the microbiome to weight loss. Then you'll get to the microbiome diet plan, which I designed with the science in mind. The two-phase meal plan is designed to repair and restore your microbiome. In just six weeks, you'll find yourself on the path to sustained weight loss, but the microbiome diet is about more than just that. You have the potential for better digestion, more energy, and better-quality sleep. Following this plan will help you improve your overall health and feel great while doing it.

You'll have everything you need to get started: six weeks of menus, shopping lists, more than 120 easy-to-follow and affordable recipes, and plenty of preparation tips. Because I know that no one has time to cook three meals a day, I've included plenty of grab-and-go meals, and lots of options to make good use of leftovers. However, you shouldn't stop at the end of the six weeks. The meal plan is designed to provide guidance as you transition to a healthier way of eating, but there are enough varied and tasty recipes in this book to keep you and your loved ones eating healthy and supporting your microbiomes for a lifetime.

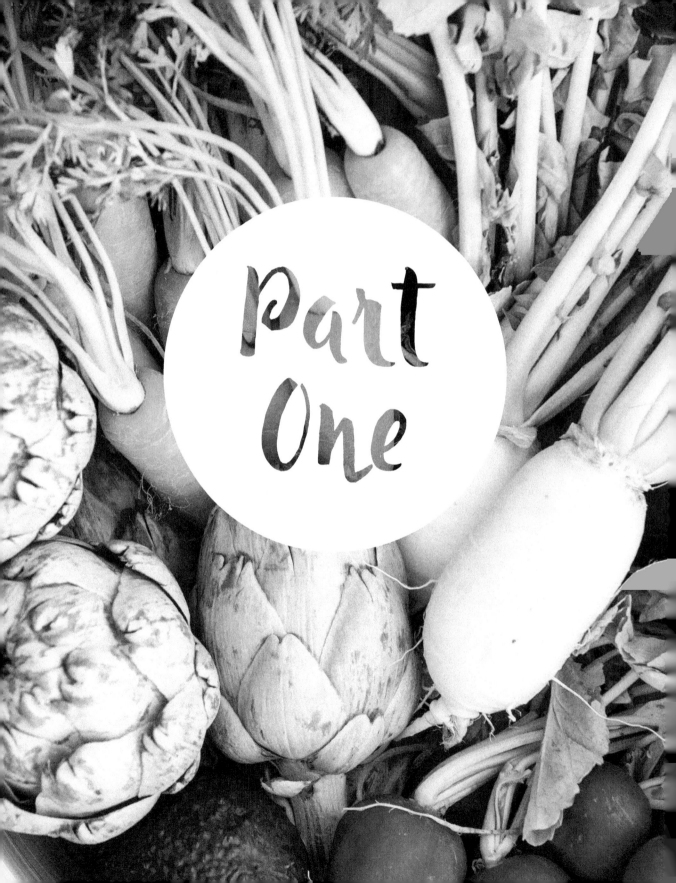

Part
One

Your Microbiome Diet Primer

Before we jump into the meal plan, let's take some time to get to know and understand the principles of the microbiome diet. The bottom line is this: You have the power to improve your health by optimizing your gut bacteria. I am going to guide you through the basics of the diet so you will understand the concepts, which will make the diet easier to follow. I want it to feel so natural that you forget you are on a "diet" at all. First, here's the lowdown on what microbiomes are and why they are so important to your health, weight, and well-being.

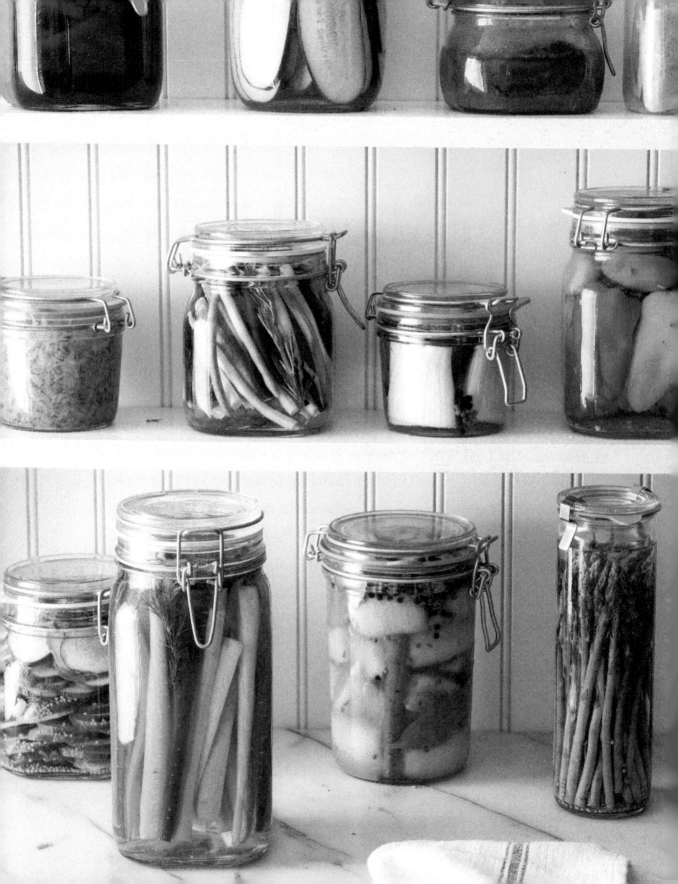

The Microbiome and You

There has been a dramatic rise of interest in the human microbiome in recent years, and as a result, the amount of research on the topic has grown exponentially. New scientific methods that allow us to do research more quickly have been a contributing factor. Growing interest from the public has been a large component in the expansion of the field as well. A substantial reason for the surge of interest is the promising link between the microbiome and health, with the suggestion that we have the power to make beneficial changes to our own well-being by encouraging a healthy microbiome. Before we get to how and what to eat to support the microbiome, it's important to take a closer look at the role the microbiome plays in weight loss and promoting a healthier you.

Getting to Know Your Microbiome

The microbiome is a collection of microorganisms that exist in staggering numbers; in fact, there are more microorganisms in the microbiome than we have human cells. When scientists started defining the microbiome, *microbiota* was the term they used to talk about the collection of microorganisms, and *microbiome* was what they called the genetic material of those organisms. We use these terms more loosely now.

Scientific research suggests that what we eat affects the profile of the bacteria (the microbes) in our guts. What goes on with our microbes affects our guts, and what goes on in our guts has enormous health implications. Research also suggests that any changes in the microbiome happen extremely quickly—in a matter of days. Because shifts can happen in detrimental as well as beneficial ways, it is important to consider what we put into our microbiomes on a daily basis. This is a plan for a lifetime.

Remember when unlocking the human genome was going to make it possible to solve all our problems . . . but didn't? Well, there was a factor at play that the researchers didn't take into account: the microbiome. With more advanced research tools, they are now uncovering a whole new set of potential interventions.

WHAT DOES HEALTHY LOOK LIKE?

The first step in getting to know your microbiome is learning what makes for a "healthy" microbiome. Even though we are still a way off from even knowing if there is a perfect microbiome, we can look at studies that compare the microbiomes of healthy and diseased individuals and draw some insights. The microbiomes of two individuals are wildly different, even though both may be perfectly healthy. A "healthy" microbiome is a microbiome in a person who is free of disease, within a normal weight range, and has a properly functioning digestive system.

We don't yet know enough to customize a microbiome to be "healthy," but we do know some dietary factors that improve health and digestion. Another thing we know is that we want a variety of different types of organisms. The commonality among healthy people is not the specific composition of the microbes in their guts, but that their microbiomes all have *diverse* populations of microbes.

Eating high-fiber foods is associated with a microbiome that is more diverse compared to eating a low-fiber diet. A low-fiber diet that is high in saturated fat and refined sugars reduces the microbial diversity.

THE BENEFITS OF SYMBIOSIS

Symbiosis is a mutually beneficial relationship between two organisms. In optimal health, we have a symbiotic relationship with our microbes: They are good for us and we are good for them. These are some of the benefits of being friendly neighbors:

» **Protection from pathogens**: We have established that microorganisms have a large presence in our guts, and that means that they truly are in residence, in extraordinary numbers. They help us by taking up space: They actually physically block pathogens from hanging out and making us sick. They also change the environment in the gut by making it more acidic and therefore inhospitable to invaders.

» **Extraction of nutrients and energy from our diets**: When we eat probiotic foods, some of the microbes that we ingest are transient, just hanging out for a while before being excreted. Others stick around for longer. Eating prebiotic foods feeds the microbes that have taken up longer-term residence. In the foods we eat, there are nutrients that human cells cannot digest, but our microbial neighbors can. They can use their enzymes to extract nutrients from food that we would not normally be able to break down and make vitamins that we are then able to use.

» **Contribution to normal immune function**: Our guts' microbes interact with our immune systems and play a critical role in regulating immune function. In fact, microbes can activate the gastrointestinal tract's own immune system, which is called gut-associated lymphoid tissue (GALT).

» **Production of short-chain fatty acids**: An important function of gut microbes is the ability to metabolize complex carbohydrates via fermentation to produce short-chain fatty acids (SCFA), which are a primary energy source for the cells that line our intestinal walls. Maintaining the integrity of our intestines by keeping those cells in good shape is paramount to digestive health.

FACTORS THAT INFLUENCE YOUR GUT HEALTH

» **Diet**: Diet is one of the most important factors when it comes to influencing your gut health. What you eat can initiate changes to your microbiome and those changes can happen overnight—literally. Studies show that significant changes can occur in the profile of your gut bacteria in as little as 24 hours. Diet is the factor over which you have the most control when making changes to affect your health.

» **Antibiotics**: While antibiotics can absolutely be necessary and even lifesaving, they are also often prescribed in cases where they are not needed. When you take a course of antibiotics, you are wiping out the good bacteria along with the bad and therefore disrupting your microbial ecosystem.

» **Childbirth**: Before birth, a fetus is germ-free; it is not until delivery that a child is either inoculated with the mother's vaginal bacteria or, in the case of a Cesarean section, the environmental bacteria of the room. Because there is evidence that vaginal childbirth is preferential for the infant microbiome, there is inquiry into the potential benefit of swabbing newborns born via C-section with the mother's bacteria.

» **Breastfeeding**: Looking at the microbiome of infants who are formula-fed versus those who are breast-fed reveals significant differences. Breast-fed babies have a bacterial composition that some research suggests might lead to a reduced risk of obesity and atopic disease (allergies). Breast milk contains sugars that feed the microbes in the infant's gut.

» **Age**: Before you are born, you are free of microbes entirely. During the first two years of life, your gut bacteria develops and becomes more stable, remaining in that stable state throughout most of your life. As you approach your older years, your microbiome shifts again to become less diverse.

What Is Dysbiosis?

The term *dysbiosis* describes a microbial imbalance that often manifests within the large microbial community in our guts. The theory is that when things in our guts are out of whack, they can have negative consequences on our body, weight, and even mood. When we speak of dysbiosis, generally we are not talking about a specific pathogen (*E. coli* or salmonella, for example) but rather an underlying disruption of the microbial ecosystem that can cause consequences for the bodily systems. The trouble with this concept is that it is vague, and because there is no underlying pathogen, it is difficult to pinpoint a precise definition. We cannot (yet) look at the ecosystem of an individual's microorganisms and make a diagnosis. Although dysbiosis is a major buzzword, it is unfortunately not yet a meaningful one in practical terms. However, there are some health conditions that have been linked to disruptive changes in the microbial community in the gut.

HEALTH CONDITIONS LINKED TO DAMAGED GUT MICROBES

Many health problems have been linked to gut microbes. In general, we do not yet know what to make of, or if there is a way to treat, the microbiomes of unhealthy patients. The first step is to understand what the differences are in the microbiomes of healthy and sick individuals, then see if we can establish patterns to use as diagnostic tools.

» **Allergies and asthma**: The gut microbes in those with allergies and asthma tend to be different from those without these conditions. This difference is probably something that is established early on in life, during the formative years of the microbiome.

» **Colorectal cancer**: Though there are many factors at play in colorectal cancer, there are measurable microbial changes that occur in patients' gut bacteria.

» **Diabetes**: The gut microbiome appears to play a role in blood sugar regulation. Studying changes to gut bacteria in the context of understanding diabetes is a promising new area of study.

» **Inflammatory bowel disease (IBD)**: Crohn's Disease and ulcerative colitis are both forms of IBD that have been linked to changes in the microbiome.

» **Irritable bowel syndrome (IBS)**: Symptoms of IBS can include pain, diarrhea, or constipation. Looking at changes to the gut microbes in IBS patients is an emerging line of inquiry. The potential for identifying subtypes of IBS and accompanying treatments are on the horizon.

» **Obesity**: The types of bacteria that predominate the microbiomes of obese individuals differ starkly from those in the microbiome of normal-weight people. While there are many factors associated with obesity, the type of gut bacteria may be an important factor because certain microbes are better at extracting calories from our food.

» **Small Intestinal Bacterial Overgrowth (SIBO)**: In SIBO, bacteria from the large intestine is translocated to the small intestine. Although the bacteria aren't necessarily pathogenic (disease-causing), they are in excess and in the wrong location. An overabundance of bacteria in the small intestine can cause symptoms ranging from gas, bloating, constipation, or diarrhea to poor absorption of vitamins.

Symptoms of Gut Disruption

Many conditions have been associated with disruptions in the microbiome. There are also several common symptoms of gut disruption within an imbalanced microbiome. If you experience one or more symptom in the following list, you may benefit from some dietary intervention.

Anxiety: Preliminary studies in animals have shown that your gut health can have a correlation with your brain health. Giving animals probiotics (supplements containing beneficial strains of bacteria) has been shown to reduce their anxiety.

Constipation: Commonly caused by a lack of high-fiber food choices, constipation can be a sign that your microbes are not functioning optimally.

Diarrhea: A sign that your food is not being digested well is diarrhea. This could be caused by a specific pathogen or dietary intolerance, both of which are modulated by gut bacteria.

Difficulty losing weight: Normal-weight and overweight individuals appear to have different microbe profiles in their guts. We can dream of the potential for skinny-bug transplants one day!

Eczema and acne: Eruptions on the skin could be related to disruptions in the gut. There is even some emerging evidence that using probiotics topically on the skin can be a treatment for dermatological concerns.

Gas and bloating: Your gut's bug buddies are keen on fermentation, so gas and bloating can be a sign that your bugs are working. However, in excess it can mean that something is off.

The Microbiome and Your Weight

The best way to address the connection of the microbiome to weight is by looking directly at the research. Dr. Jeffrey Gordon led a groundbreaking study in which gut bacteria from human twins were transplanted into germ-free mice. Germ-free mice are mice that have been raised without any exposure to bacteria and are considered devoid of a microbiome, making them perfect subjects for this type of experiment. The twist with this experiment was that in each of the pairs of human twins, one twin was obese, and one twin was lean. The remarkable result: When the human gut bacteria were transplanted into the mice, the mice that received the bacteria from the obese twins became obese, and the mice that received the bacteria from the thin twins stayed thin!

Then the researchers changed the diets of the mice to see what happened. They found that when they put both the lean and the obese mice on a low-fat diet, the obese mice got thin. A striking thing is that regardless of diet, the thin mice did not get obese. This is a very encouraging result (at least in mice): The lean stayed lean, and the obese could get lean by changing their diets. But this only happened when the mice were given food that was low in fat and high in fruits and vegetables. When the experiment was repeated with mouse food that mimicked the standard American diet (SAD), which is high in fat and low in fruits and vegetables, the fat mice stayed fat.

We have to remember that the study began with human bacteria transplanted into mice, so we are talking about changes occurring in mice, not humans. As encouraging as it would be to assume that the same could happen to people, we just do not know yet. However, it does give us some solid evidence that the composition of the microbiome may play a big part in determining whether someone is obese or normal weight.

We can hope the principle holds true in humans: that given the proper diet, you could lose weight and shift your microbiome to a lean profile, where it would stay as long as you stayed on the diet. Even though we don't have an elegant study to demonstrate this in humans yet, we do know that changes in the microbiome occur very quickly, and we know the foods that lean people are eating. The diet plan in this book is designed to help you put these "skinny bugs" to work.

Food and Your Microbiome

As we have discussed, there are multiple factors that influence the condition of your microbiome, but many of those are out of our control. Unfortunately, we can't turn back time and make sure that we all avoid being born via C-section and that we are exclusively breast-fed. We do know, however, that the food you eat directly impacts your microbiome health. The foods that make up the SAD diet (lots of refined low-fiber carbohydrates and saturated fats from fried food and meats) are enemies to your healthy gut flora. Conversely, food choices like high-fiber carbohydrates (whole grains, legumes, nuts, and seeds) help feed a healthy microbiome.

What you eat can play a vital role in shaping the microbe population in your gut. Microbes themselves and nourishment for microbes can be an important part of the diet as well. Let's now take a closer look at prebiotics and probiotics and how they influence your microbiome health.

PREBIOTICS

Fast food for your gut microbes! Prebiotics are foods that the microbes in your gut love to eat—because, yes, they need to be nourished as well. We want to keep our microbes happy and that means feeding them their favorite foods.

To be classified as prebiotic, a food must meet certain criteria. They must:

» be a nondigestible food ingredient (a fiber that our human cells cannot break down)

» affect the host in a beneficial way

» selectively stimulate the growth and/or activity of bacteria in the colon

Although prebiotics may sound like an entirely new concept, they are found in foods that you likely already enjoy. Bananas, whole grains, asparagus, and honey are just a few examples. To get a little more technical, prebiotics are nonstarch poly-saccharides and oligosaccharides (a mouthful!) that are contained in foods and also food additives: fructo-oligosaccharides, inulin, and lactulose.

What foods are they in?

» **Fruits**: bananas, melons

» **Legumes**: black beans, chickpeas, kidney beans, lentils

» **Vegetables**: asparagus, chicory root, garlic, sunchokes (Jerusalem artichokes), leeks, onions, shallots,

» **Whole grains**: whole wheat

Although prebiotics are a gut superfood, they can trigger symptoms in people with IBS (10 to 15 percent of the population). Because by definition prebiotics are short-chain carbohydrates that are easily fermentable, they can lead to excessive gas, bloating, constipation, or diarrhea. If you find that prebiotic foods are causing disagreeable symptoms, you may want to investigate following a low-FODMAP diet (a diet low in fermentable carbohydrates) to help identify your triggers. Prebiotics feed your microbes, so you do not want to eliminate them entirely; it is therefore important to figure out your tolerance so you can enjoy as wide a variety of foods as possible.

PROBIOTICS

According to the World Health Organization, the definition of a probiotic is a live microorganism (live bacteria) that when ingested in adequate amounts confers health benefits to the host. It is relevant then to note that, based on this definition, cultured and fermented foods are not necessarily "probiotic," because each and every bottle of miso is not tested in a lab to see if it can treat a specific health problem. So, strictly speaking, the term *probiotic* should be reserved for live microbes that have been shown in controlled human studies to impart a specific health benefit (i.e., a particular strain of bacteria helps lower cholesterol). Despite efforts to reserve the term for that specific meaning, the word *probiotic* has come to be synonymous with both fermented foods and supplements. Although we are not yet able to be prescriptive (meaning we can't yet say "eat this yogurt for this condition"), we do know that fermented foods with live and active cultures have healthy belly benefits.

The benefits of eating probiotics line up exactly with the list of incredible functions of the microbiome. Coincidence? Not really—because your microbiome is your collection of microbes, and probiotics are microbes too. Although we are ingesting them, studies have shown that probiotics tend not to stick around for the long term. Nonetheless, even as transients they are beneficial. Plus, their transience is all the more reason to make them a regular staple in your diet.

Probiotic foods you can find at the grocery store:

» Buttermilk

» Kefir (coconut, dairy, water)

» Kimchi

» Kombucha

» Miso

» Pickles (not made with vinegar, unpasteurized)

» Sauerkraut (not made with vinegar, unpasteurized)

» Tempeh

» Yogurt (almond, coconut, dairy, soy)

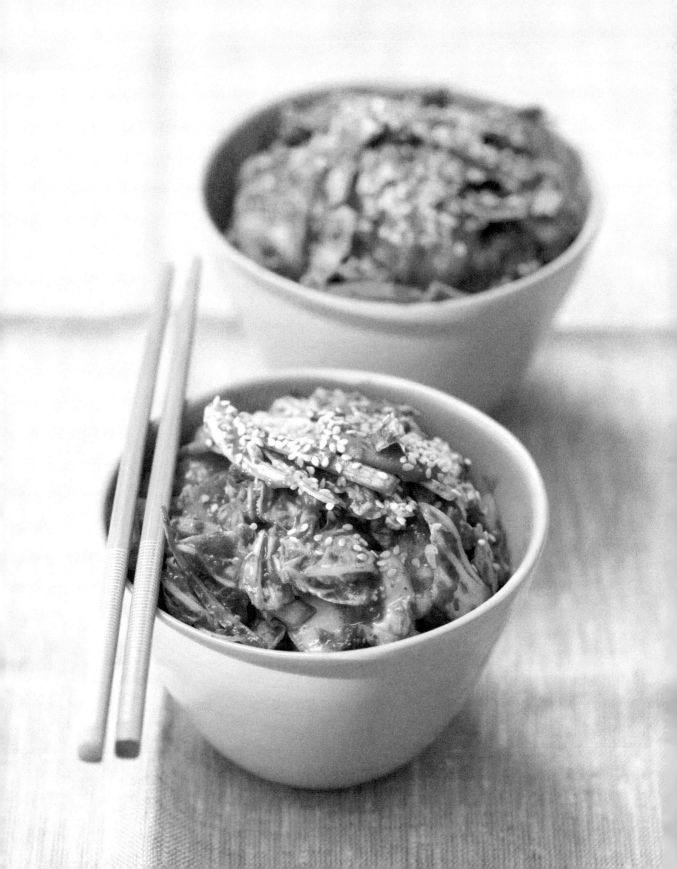

The Microbiome Diet

Now that we've reviewed the important role the microbiome plays in maintaining your health and weight, let's take a closer look at how you should eat in order to promote a healthy microbiome. Even though we are calling this the microbiome diet, there are no hard-and-fast diet guidelines that are widely accepted. Instead, there is a large body of research. This book is inspired and influenced by the work of many different experts, notably my mentor Dr. Gerard E. Mullin, and also Dr. Jeffrey Gordon, Dr. Peter Turnbaugh, Dr. Ruth Ley, Drs. Justin and Erica Sonnenburg, Dr. Robynne Chutkan, and others, who have made contributions to the field of research and who are also spreading the word to the public, which is instrumental in raising awareness that we can improve our health by improving our microbiomes.

The Guidelines

Studies involving the microbiome are new, and the science behind how certain foods influence your health often changes, as can be seen from the many books available that promote very different ideas about how to eat to support your gut health. Here, I try to keep things straightforward, approachable, and based on the current science. You'll learn about the general common principles that are supported by scientific literature.

CHOOSE HIGH-FIBER CARBS

Fiber does the double duty of sweeping your intestines clean and keeping things moving regularly. Fiber also slows down digestion, which keeps us full longer, a boon when you are trying to shed pounds. Fiber is found in carbohydrates so we don't want to avoid carbohydrates altogether. Instead, we should choose higher-fiber sources like whole grains, legumes, fruits, and vegetables.

EAT MORE PLANTS

Plants are full of fiber in addition to vitamins and minerals that we need to support our microbiome. Plus, the microbes that live in your gut love to eat plants—plants are one of their favorite foods, and you want to make sure your neighbors are happy, right? Our microbes need nourishment just like we do, and we want to provide them with the healthiest foods possible so they will thrive and in turn help us thrive.

FERMENT YOUR FOODS

Probiotics are superfoods for your gut. One of the best ways to make sure you are supporting your microbiome is to add new friends (by eating probiotic foods) to live among your microbes (even if they don't hang out forever). One affordable and surprisingly easy way to do this is by fermenting foods yourself. Some of the healthiest fermented foods are vegetables, such as real probiotic pickles. Another category that is often overlooked is fermented drinks, such as kombucha.

LIMIT YOUR MEAT INTAKE

Often when people think "diet," they believe the answer to losing weight is more protein. That can be true, but it is important to think about the source of your protein. Studies have shown that red meat can have serious negative consequences on the microbiome and, as a result, on the health of your heart. While it is important to eat all the macronutrients, we want to make sure we get good protein from plant foods.

The theory is that red meat delivers L-carnitine to your gut bacteria. These gut microbes digest the L-carnitine and turn it into a compound called trimethylamine-N-oxide (TMAO). In studies conducted in mice, TMAO has been shown to cause clogged arteries.

AVOID GLUTEN

Gluten is a protein found in whole and refined grains. Gluten also hides out in unexpected places, like sauces and marinades, because it is frequently used as a preservative. Although we do not know if gluten is particularly detrimental to the microbiome, I have excluded it from this diet plan with the goal of weight loss in mind. I also exclude gluten because when gluten is added to a sauce or marinade, there are usually lots of other additives in that item that you should be avoiding. We all react to gluten differently, so if you don't feel sensitive to gluten, feel free to reintroduce whole grains containing gluten back into your diet in limited quantities after you've worked your way through the six-week plan.

AVOID SUGAR AND SUGAR SUBSTITUTES

It is pretty well established that sugar does not support health. It leads to blood sugar spikes and weight gain, which over the long term can have serious health consequences, including type 2 diabetes. One way that people meet their sweet cravings without the accompanying calories is by using artificial sweeteners. Unfortunately, the research shows that sugar substitutes can affect the microbiome in such a way that they can still cause diabetes. Let's make sure we satisfy our desires for sweetness in healthier ways, for example, with fruit or small amounts of honey or maple syrup.

CHOOSE CULTURED DAIRY

Dairy as a category has gotten an unfairly negative reputation. You will find a lot of inconsistency in dairy guidelines within other microbiome diets, which suggests that there is no hard-and-fast rule. In this book, I am recommending emphasizing cultured dairy products. You will find that some of the recipes included here use cheese and cultured probiotic dairy products, but not milk.

AVOID FOOD ADDITIVES

In recent years, health concerns have fueled a real evolution in the types of foods that we eat. Nondairy milk, such as almond milk, for example, has become extremely popular, which is fantastic for those who are looking to avoid dairy. In order to make the "milk" have a desirable consistency, however, additives are often included, some of which, notably carrageenan, carboxymethylcellulose, and Polysorbate 80, have been shown to have negative consequences on the integrity of the gut lining and the gut microbiome. So when it comes to foods, keep the ingredient list short. That doesn't mean avoiding almond milk completely, it just means checking the labels.

LIMIT ALCOHOL INTAKE

Alcohol, though not off-limits, should be consumed in moderation during your six-week meal plan and beyond. Choose heart-healthy beverages, such as red wine, and consume no more than 1 to 2 glasses of wine 2 to 3 times a week. Consuming alcohol in excess has been proven to negatively alter gut microbiota.

A Two-Phase Plan

The microbiome diet meal plan is based on two distinct phases. The first phase will be a little bit more restrictive to give your gut a reset. We want to make sure your gut is in tip-top shape in preparation for the second phase, which will help you sustain all the beneficial changes you made in phase one. Although this plan is designed for a total time frame of six weeks, it is intended to support your microbiome well beyond that— you can continue in phase two for as long as you'd like (the longer the better!) and reference this book and its recipes on an ongoing basis. Here are some more details about each phase:

PHASE ONE

Restore. For the first three weeks of this diet plan, you're going to repair your gut microbiome. The way you're going to do that is by removing the foods that are damaging it with their bad bacteria. The goal of this phase is to reduce distressing digestive symptoms so your gut can heal. We want you to be feeling great so that you're ready for phase two.

PHASE TWO

Sustain. For the second three-week period, your goal is to rebalance the gut flora and reestablish a healthy microbiome. You will see that the rules are a bit more liberal, and the diet is based on whole foods that are delicious and simple to prepare. This is because the second phase is going to become your new normal.

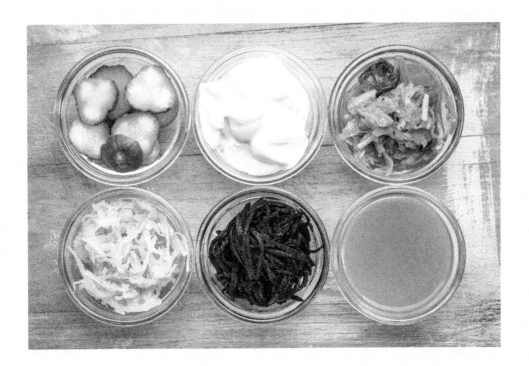

Supplements—Do You Really Need Them?

When you read books about the microbiome, you might find yourself sifting through overwhelming lists of supplements. Not to say that those books are wrong; there are conditions when supplements can be helpful, but following those recommendations can end up being very expensive. The good news is that current scientific research tells us you can optimize your diet to support a healthy life with a healthy microbiome without having to buy anything you can't find at the grocery store. I don't recommend store-bought supplements to everyone (though further scientific research may contradict me someday!), rather you should be getting your daily dose of microbes through your diet. It can be useful to take probiotics at certain times. For instance, if you're taking a course of antibiotics, it is important to space out the doses so the antibiotics don't kill the good bugs too. But in general, you can forget about those expensive supplements and keep your costs down by incorporating probiotic foods into your diet.

Phase One Microbiome Diet Plan

What to Eat?

After all the buildup, you probably just want to know what to eat! Phase one is full of whole foods and healthy foods. It is more restrictive, but that is because, as already described, you want to reset your gut, leaving it calm and healed. It will be well worth the effort. In this phase you'll remove all processed and packaged foods, meat, gluten, sugars, artificial sweeteners, and food-additive stabilizers. Instead of those unhealthy choices, you can enjoy lots of high-fiber vegetables and fermented vegetables, gluten-free whole grains, fruits, nuts, and legumes. Limited quantities of seafood can also be enjoyed, as well as limited amounts of cultured dairy and eggs.

Use this handy chart to see which foods to choose and which foods to lose during phase one.

MICROBIOME PRINCIPLE
Fermented Foods and Drinks

CHOOSE	LOSE
Fermented vegetables such as fermented pickles, kimchi, miso, and sauerkraut	**Vinegar-based foods** such as certain types of pickles and sauerkraut
Fermented drinks such as kombucha	**Processed dairy** such as milk
Fermented dairy such as kefir and yogurt	

MICROBIOME PRINCIPLE
No Added Sugar

CHOOSE	LOSE
Fruit, if you're craving something sweet	**All added sugar** such as brown and white sugar, high fructose corn syrup, honey, maple syrup, and sugar substitutes

Plant Strong/High-Fiber Carbohydrates

CHOOSE

Fruits (frozen okay) such as apples, avocados, bananas, berries, cherries, citrus, coconut, figs, grapes, mangos, melons, oranges, and pears

Legumes such as beans, chickpeas, lentils, lima beans, and split peas

Nuts and seeds such as almonds, chia, flaxseed, quinoa, and walnuts

Vegetables (frozen okay) such as artichokes, asparagus, beets, broccoli, carrots, cabbage, cauliflower, green beans, kale, okra, onions, parsnips, peas, peppers, potatoes, spinach, tomatoes, and turnips

Whole grains such as amaranth, brown and wild rice, millet, oats (gluten-free), and quinoa

LOSE

Meat, especially processed meats like bacon, ham, hot dogs, processed cold cuts, and sausage

Processed carbohydrates such as boxed cereal, bread, highly processed grains, white rice, and waffles

Processed fruits such as canned fruits in sugar

Whole grains containing gluten such as barley, bulgar wheat, and farro

MICROBIOME PRINCIPLE

Eliminate Additives

CHOOSE

Unprocessed foods without additives such as fresh fruits and vegetables, nuts and seeds

LOSE

Foods containing additives such as artificial sweeteners, carboxymethylcellulose carrageenan, and Polysorbate 80

TIP Limit cooking fermented foods (probiotics are living and can be killed by high temperatures).

Phase Two Microbiome Diet Plan

What to Eat?

Phase two is designed to sustain the positive changes that you made during phase one. During this three-week phase, you'll continue to enjoy the foods you've been eating in phase one, but you'll also reintroduce some foods, such as small amounts of beef, pork, and chicken, as well as honey, and maple syrup. Remember to be mindful of any changes in how you feel as you reintroduce foods that you have not had in some time.

MICROBIOME PRINCIPLE

Fermented Foods and Drinks

CHOOSE

Fermented vegetables such as fermented pickles, kimchi, miso, and sauerkraut

Fermented drinks such as kombucha

Cultured dairy like kefir and yogurt

LOSE

Vinegar-based foods such as certain types of pickles and sauerkraut

MICROBIOME PRINCIPLE

No Added Sugar

CHOOSE

Naturally sweet foods such as fruit, limited honey, and maple syrup

LOSE

All added sugar such as brown and white sugar, and high fructose corn syrup

Plant Strong/High-Fiber Carbohydrates

CHOOSE

Fruits (frozen okay) such as apples, avocados, bananas, berries, cherries, citrus, coconut, figs, grapes, mangos, melons, oranges, and pears

Legumes such as beans, chickpeas, lentils, lima beans, and split peas

Nuts and seeds such as almonds, chia, flaxseed, quinoa, and walnuts

Vegetables (frozen okay) such as artichokes, asparagus, beets, broccoli, carrots, cabbage, cauliflower, green beans, kale, okra, onions, parsnips, peas, peppers, potatoes, spinach, tomatoes, and turnips

Whole grains such as amaranth, brown and wild rice, millet, oats (gluten-free), and quinoa

LOSE

Highly processed foods such as processed grains like white rice

Processed fruits such as canned fruits in sugar

Processed meats such as bacon, ham, hot dogs, processed cold cuts, sausage, and large portions of all meats/multiple portions of meat per day

Eliminate Additives

CHOOSE

Unprocessed foods without additives such as fresh fruits and vegetables, nuts and seeds

LOSE

Foods containing additives such as artificial sweeteners, carboxymethylcellulose carrageenan, and Polysorbate 80

TIP Limit cooking fermented foods (probiotics are living and can be killed by high temperatures).

Home Fermentation 101

Home fermentation is surprisingly simple to do. People have been fermenting foods around the world for hundreds of years, and most often they have done it in kitchens lacking the modern amenities you have in yours. Instead of spending loads of money on store-bought ferments, try your hand at this time-tested craft to save big on your grocery bill, and have a bit of fun in the process.

To ferment fruits and vegetables, you need little specialized equipment; a fermentation vessel is where all the magic happens and is a necessary tool. However, if you have a couple of pint- or quart-size mason jars, you are all set, especially for the projects in this book. Glass is most preferable for fermentation, as it is easily accessible and usually inexpensive. Stoneware fermentation crocks and food-grade plastic containers can also be used when you are ready to scale up, but are not necessary for these small-scale ferments.

Any utensil or bowl that you use for fermentation should be made of non-reactive materials, such as stainless steel, glass, or ceramic, as the salt used in many fermentation recipes can react with metals. Enameled metal bowls and pots in theory would work, but tiny cracks can allow for reactions between salt and metal, and therefore, they should be avoided. A couple of plastic lids for mason jars are also great for storage and prevent the rusting that can occur when using metal lids and rings.

Most of the fermenting recipes in this book call for sea salt. Salt protects against unwanted microbial growth during fermentation and is an integral part of the process. Sea salt is widely available and a great choice for fermenting. The most important thing when selecting a salt is to make sure it does not contain any iodine or additional additives, which are used in table salt to prevent caking but can cause problems in fermentation. Canning and pickling salt can be substituted for sea salt, but avoid using any sea salts that are not white, as they can too adversely affect fermentation.

Before beginning any project, be sure to wash your hands and all containers, bowls, and utensils well with warm, soapy water. Avoid using antibacterial soaps, as these can kill the good bacteria as well as the bad. Always wash utensils and your hands before you check on any ferments, and be sure to store the ferments in a location out of direct light, away from a heat source, and in plain sight, so that you do not forget about them in a cupboard during fermentation.

Tips for Success

» **Plan meals ahead of time**: This book saves you time by giving you a meal plan and shopping list for each of the six weeks.

» **Customize the diet**: I've included extra recipes that are not specifically part of the plan, so you can always swap out a meal here and there to suit your preferences. You have no excuses not to stick to the diet, even if you hate tomatoes!

» **Don't skip meals**: Eating regularly throughout the day helps stabilize your blood sugar levels and keeps your energy level even. Making the best food choices is much easier if you aren't hungry.

» **Don't skip meals before a big outing**: It is especially true that you should not skip a meal if you are going to a big event. You won't be able to resist temptation if you show up with an empty stomach.

» **Snack**: Don't ignore snacks. If you normally power through the day without stopping for a snack, that is fine, but if your energy tends to dip, make sure you eat a few snacks throughout the day to keep you feeling strong.

» **Try new recipes**: You don't have to be a chef to make the recipes included in this book. They're designed to be simple to prepare. You'll probably try some new foods that will make you feel great.

» **Get potluck-y**: If you go to a friend's or family member's for a potluck, you can bring one of your new creations. Not only will they be impressed, but you'll feel good knowing that you have something tasty and healthy to eat.

» **Don't fear dining out**: Try to look up the menu of a restaurant online so you can plan your meal before you get to the restaurant. You will feel much more relaxed when you go to order and will make fewer impulsive choices.

» **Take notes**: You are making some big changes and it may help if you keep a record of what you are eating. Journaling your food intake can help you stay accountable, help you notice changes in how you feel, or track how much weight you are losing!

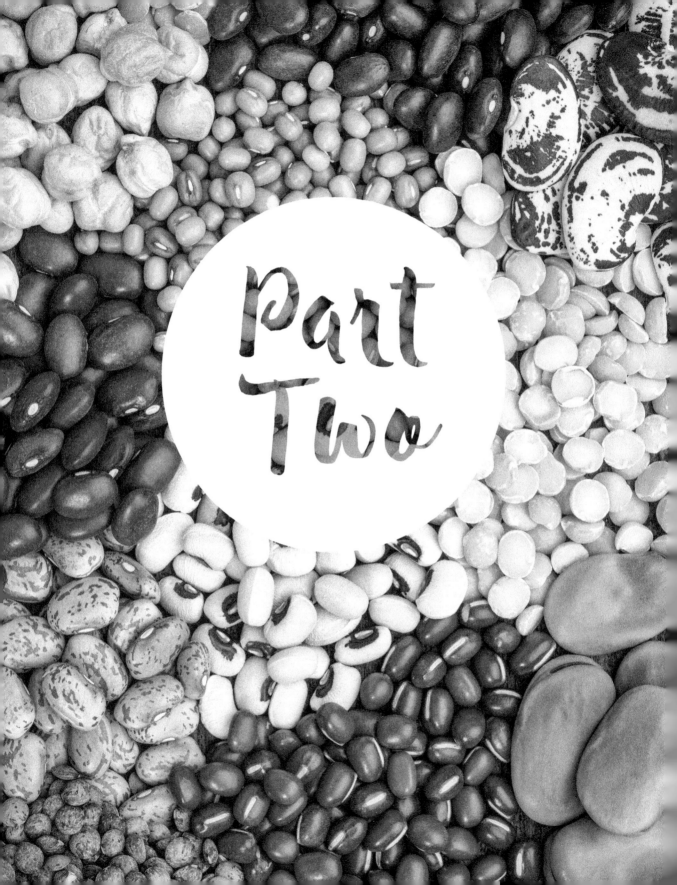

Part
Two

The Meal Plan

This meal plan takes the guesswork out of cooking for the microbiome diet, giving you three meals a day and offering ten snack options each week that you can pick and choose from. Swap in one of the extra recipes if something in the meal plan doesn't appeal to you. Most of us are too busy to cook three meals a day, so there are grab-and-go breakfasts and lunches, and lots of opportunities to make good use of leftovers. You'll also find plenty of tips on how to prepare food ahead of time to make your life easier. Remember, stress is a negative contributor to the microbiome—I want you to stay calm in the kitchen!

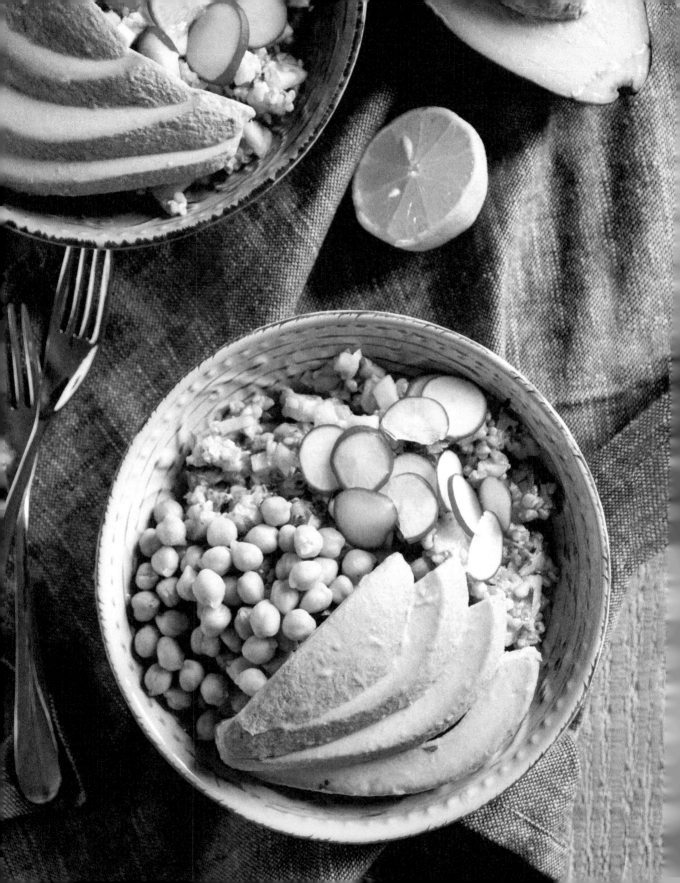

Phase One Meal Plan
Restore

The first phase of the microbiome diet is designed to restore your microbes to their happy place. Although phase one is more restrictive, the entire diet is designed to feel manageable. The main difference you will notice is that there is no meat. There are also no manufactured carbohydrates, such as bread. This transition may be challenging, but it will be worth it.

Week One

The first week may be the toughest, because you will be making some significant changes to the way you eat, but it will also be an exciting week. It may be a little early to see any major payoff, but you will start to notice a difference in how you feel, and you might even lose a pound or two. You may feel moody, irritable, or tired as you come off sugar; this is a natural reaction. Your body is adjusting after being hooked on sugar. It will take a few days to rebound, but you will feel so much better afterward. Take a look at the Get Ahead sidebars for suggestions for what you can do to prepare for the week ahead. Don't let the long pantry list intimidate you; you won't need to replenish the pantry every week. Plus, you may find that you already have many of these items at home.

SNACKS TO ENJOY:

- Handful of almonds
- Hardboiled egg with salt and pepper
- Clementine or satsuma orange
- Sweet Potato Chips (page 186)
- Handful of fresh blueberries or raspberries
- ½ cup unsweetened applesauce
- Celery sticks with hummus
- Handful of granola (Beware of added sugars in store-bought granola—see recipe for Oat, Walnut, and Golden Raisin Granola on page 85)
- Leftover Simple Green Side Salad (page 107)
- Yogurt with Fermented Raspberry Chia Jam (page 218)

Week One Shopping List

CANNED / BOTTLED / PACKAGED FOODS

Applesauce, unsweetened
(1 [24-ounce] jar)
Black beans, low-sodium
(4 [15-ounce] cans)
Coconut milk, light
(1 [15-ounce] can)
Fermented vegetables
(1 [16-ounce] jar or
make them yourself—
see chapter 12)
Kalamata olives
(1 [9-ounce] jar)
Tomatoes, whole, low-sodium
(2 [28-ounce] cans)
Tuna, packed in water
(1 [6-ounce] can)
Vegetable broth, low-sodium
(2 [32-ounce] containers)

DAIRY AND EGGS

Feta cheese, crumbled
(4 ounces)
Kefir, plain (1 quart, or make
your own—see page 211)
Large eggs (1 dozen plus
1 half dozen)
Parmesan cheese, shredded
(4 ounces)
Yogurt, plain, unsweetened
(1 quart)

FROZEN FOODS

Blackberries, whole
(16 ounces)
Corn kernels (16 ounces)
Mango, chunks (16 ounces)

PANTRY STAPLES

Almond flour
Almonds, sliced
Baking powder
Black pepper
Cayenne pepper, ground
Chia seeds
Cinnamon, ground
Coriander, ground
Cumin, ground
Dill, dried
Flaxseed, whole
Flaxseed meal
Garlic powder
Ginger, ground
Ketchup (Or make it yourself—
see page 199)
Lentils, French green
Mustard seeds, whole
Mustard, whole-grain
Nonstick cooking spray
Oats, rolled, gluten-free
Oil, extra-virgin olive
Oil, canola
Oil, coconut
Oil, sesame, toasted
Onion powder
Quinoa
Raisins, golden
Salt
Sesame seeds
Tamari
Turmeric, ground
Vanilla extract
Vinegar, balsamic
Vinegar, rice
Vinegar, white wine
Walnut pieces

MEAT AND SEAFOOD

Cod fillets (1 pound)
Salmon fillets (1 pound)
Tilapia fillets (1 pound)

PRODUCE

Arugula (5 ounces)
Bananas (2)
Beets (4)
Bell peppers, green (2)
Bell peppers, red (3)
Bok choy (1 head)
Blueberries (1 pint)
Carrots (4)
Cauliflower (2 heads)
Celery (1 bunch)
Cherry tomatoes (1 pint)
Chile, green (1)
Cilantro, fresh (1 bunch)
Cucumber (1)
Fennel (1 bulb)
Garlic, fresh (1 head)
Ginger, fresh (1 knob)
Honeydew melon (1)
Kale (2 bunches)
Kiwi fruit (1)
Kohlrabi (1 bulb)
Lemons (3)
Lettuce, red or green leaf
(1 head)
Lettuce, romaine (2 heads)
Mushrooms, cremini
(24 ounces)
Onions, yellow (6)
Potatoes, white (1)
Raspberries (1 pint)
Scallions (2 bunches)
Spinach, baby (10 ounces)
Tomatoes (4)

OTHER

Almond milk, plain,
unsweetened (1 pint)

Week One Meal Plan

	BREAKFAST	LUNCH	DINNER
MONDAY	Quinoa Almond Muffins (page 82) and ½ cup fresh fruit	Tuna Salad Lettuce Wraps (page 146) with ¼ cup fermented vegetables	Black Bean Veggie Burgers (page 133)
TUESDAY	Oat, Walnut, and Golden Raisin Granola (page 85) with yogurt	Arugula and Walnut Quinoa Bowl (page 121)	Italian Lentil Salad (page 127)
WEDNESDAY	Quinoa Almond Muffin (page 82) with yogurt and ½ cup fruit	Leftover Black Bean Veggie Burger and ¼ cup fermented vegetables	Simple Roasted Salmon Fillets with Tomatoes (page 147) and Asian Kale Salad with Sesame-Ginger Dressing (page 108)
THURSDAY	Chia Yogurt Melon Bowl (page 90)	Leftover Italian Lentil Salad	Simple Black Bean Soup (page 101) and Fragrant Fennel and Kohlrabi Salad (page 109)
FRIDAY	Tropical Turmeric Kefir Smoothie (page 74)	Leftover Asian Kale Salad with Sesame-Ginger Dressing and leftover Simple Black Bean Soup	Tilapia with Coconut Curry Sauce (page 151) with Cauliflower Rice (page 188) and ¼ cup fermented vegetables
SATURDAY	Poached Eggs on a Bed of Kale Pesto and Tomatoes (page 80)	Creamy Tomato Soup (page 98), Simple Green Side Salad (page 107), and ¼ cup fermented vegetables	Balsamic Mushroom and Corn Stir-Fry (page 139) with Cauliflower Rice (page 188)
SUNDAY	Make-Ahead Egg and Vegetable Cups (page 76) with Quinoa Almond Muffin (page 82)	Beet Yogurt Soup (page 95), Simple Green Side Salad (page 107), and ¼ cup fermented vegetables	Asian-Style Cod and Vegetables in Parchment (page 148)

GET AHEAD

Sunday: Make the Oat, Walnut, and Golden Raisin Granola (page 85). This is a great breakfast option to have on hand.

Cook 1 cup of dry quinoa so you have enough for the Quinoa Almond Muffins (page 82) that you are going to make today, and also for the Arugula and Walnut Quinoa Bowl (page 121).

Make the muffins and freeze four of them for use in week three.

Make the Tuna Salad Lettuce Wraps (page 146) through step 2.

Monday: Prep the Arugula and Walnut Quinoa Bowl. Place all the ingredients in a large bowl or jar without the vinegar and oil. Mix the dressing before serving.

Wednesday night: Prep the Chia Yogurt Melon Bowl (page 90).

Sunday: After making the Make-Ahead Egg and Vegetable Cups (page 76), freeze four of them to use later.

Week Two

This week, you may still be easing your way into the plan, but hopefully you are starting to adjust to the changes—and enjoying your new recipes. You may be experiencing some extra gas—that is your microbes saying hello. It is totally normal, but if you are really uncomfortable scale back on the beans. As a reminder, this meal plan incorporates leftovers to make your life easier, because, honestly, it's often not realistic to cook three meals a day. Weekday breakfasts and lunches are designed to be grab-and-go, so that should help make the transition to your healthier microbiome easier. Even though desserts are not included in the plan, if you have a sweet tooth and are having trouble staying on track, check out chapter 13 for some dessert options. If you are doing okay without it, more power to you!

SNACKS TO ENJOY:

- Handful of walnuts
- ½ cup fresh strawberries or blueberries
- Leftover Simple Green Side Salad (page 107)
- Celery stalks with nut butter
- Handful of kalamata olives
- Handful of granola (Beware of added sugars in store-bought granola—see recipe for Oat, Walnut, and Golden Raisin Granola on page 85)
- ½ cup yogurt with fresh or frozen berries
- 2 or 3 dried apricots
- Fermented Carrot Sticks (page 216)
- Fermented dill pickle

Week Two Shopping List

CANNED / BOTTLED / PACKAGED FOODS

Applesauce, unsweetened
(1 [24-ounce] jar)
Black beans, low-sodium
(3 [15-ounce] cans)
Chickpeas, low-sodium
(3 [15-ounce] cans)
Coconut milk, light
(1 [15-ounce] can)
Fermented vegetables
(1 [16-ounce] jar, or
make them yourself—
see chapter 12)
Salmon, packed in water
(1 6-ounce] can)
Vegetable broth, low-sodium
(3 [32-ounce] containers)

DAIRY AND EGGS

Goat cheese, crumbled
(4 ounces)
Large eggs (1 dozen)
Parmesan cheese, shredded
(4 ounces)
Yogurt, unsweetened, plain
(2 quarts)

PANTRY STAPLES

Apricots, dried
Almond flour
Almonds, raw
Baking powder
Black pepper
Cashews, raw
Chia seeds, whole
Coconut, dried, unsweetened
Cumin, ground

Curry powder
Flaxseed, whole
Garlic powder
Lentils, French green
Lentils, red
Mustard, whole grain
Nonstick cooking spray
Oats, rolled, gluten-free
Oil, extra-virgin olive
Oil, canola
Oil, coconut
Raisins, golden
Red pepper flakes
Salt
Tamari
Thyme, dried
Turmeric, ground
Vanilla extract
Vinegar, white wine
Walnut pieces

MEAT AND SEAFOOD

Salmon fillets (2 pounds)
Tilapia fillets (1 pound)

PRODUCE

Avocado (1)
Basil, fresh (1 bunch)
Beets (1)
Bell pepper, green (1)
Bell pepper, red (1)
Blueberries (1 pint)
Brussels sprouts (1 pound)
Carrots (3)
Cauliflower (2 heads)
Celery (1 bunch)
Chile, red (1)
Cilantro, fresh (1 bunch)

Garlic, fresh (1 head)
Ginger, fresh (1 knob)
Jalapeño pepper (1)
Kale (1 bunch)
Lemongrass (1 stalk)
Lemons (5)
Lettuce, red or green leaf
(1 head)
Lettuce, romaine (1 head)
Lime (1)
Mint, fresh (1 bunch)
Mushrooms, cremini
(18 ounces)
Onions, yellow (5)
Onion, red (1)
Parsley, fresh (1 bunch)
Parsnips (4)
Peas, snap or sweet (8 ounces)
Potato, white (1)
Radishes (1 bunch)
Rosemary, fresh (2 sprigs)
Scallions (2 bunches)
Sweet potatoes (4)
Strawberries (1 pint)
Spinach (2 bunches)
Spinach, baby (12 ounces)
Tomatoes (3)

OTHER

Miso paste, red or white
(1 [12-ounce] package)
Nutritional yeast (1 [4-ounce]
package)
Sake or dry cooking wine
(1 [300-millileter] bottle)
Tofu, firm (2 [12-ounce]
packages)
Wakame seaweed flakes
(1 [2-ounce] package)

Week Two Meal Plan

	BREAKFAST	LUNCH	DINNER
MONDAY	Apricot Nut Muffins (page 83) with softboiled egg	Simple Black Bean Soup (page 101) and ¼ cup fermented vegetables	Chickpea and Spinach Stir-Fry (page 135) with Cauliflower Rice (page 188)
TUESDAY	Oat and Nut Muesli with Raspberries (page 86) with yogurt and ½ cup fruit	Salmon Salad Lettuce Wraps (page 145) and ¼ cup fermented vegetables	Malaysian-Style Coconut Tofu and Vegetable Curry (page 137) and Cauliflower Rice (page 188)
WEDNESDAY	Yogurt Parfait (page 89)	Leftover Simple Black Bean Soup	Goat Cheese and Lentil Salad (page 128)
THURSDAY	Apricot Nut Muffin (page 83) with yogurt	Leftover Chickpea and Spinach Stir-Fry with leftover Cauliflower Rice	One-Pan Salmon, Sweet Potato, and Brussels Sprouts Bake (page 155)
FRIDAY	Blueberry Ginger Smoothie (page 72)	Leftover Malaysian-Style Coconut Tofu and Vegetable Curry and leftover Cauliflower Rice	Pan-Roasted Almond-Crusted Tilapia (page 154) with Roasted Root Vegetable Medley (page 189)
SATURDAY	Fried Eggs over Greens and Beans (page 78)	Creamy Tomato Soup (page 98) and Roasted Garlic Brussels Sprouts (page 190)	Chickpea and Avocado Buckwheat Tabbouleh (page 134) and ¼ cup fermented vegetables
SUNDAY	Make-Ahead Tofu and Vegetable Frittatas (page 77) with ½ cup fruit	Curried Lentil and Parsnip Soup (page 100) and Simple Green Side Salad (page 107)	Miso Salmon and Vegetables in Parchment (page 150) with Miso Soup with Tofu and Seaweed (page 96)

GET AHEAD

Sunday: Make the Apricot Nut Muffins (page 83), which are great for a grab-and-go breakfast throughout the week. Prepare the Oat and Nut Muesli with Raspberries (page 86). Make a batch of Simple Black Bean Soup (page 101), which, like most soups, tastes even better the next day.

Monday: Prep the Salmon Salad Lettuce Wraps (page 145) through step 2.

Tuesday: Make the Yogurt Parfait (page 89) for Wednesday's breakfast.

Sunday: After making the Make-Ahead Tofu and Vegetable Frittatas (page 77), freeze four frittatas for use in week four.

Week Three

Congratulations—you have already made it to week three, which is also the last week of phase one. You have come so far! How are you feeling? Make sure to check in with yourself as you follow the microbiome diet plan. Are you enjoying the meal plans, and do you find them convenient? If you find that you like some meals more than others, you can swap them out with any of the other recipes in phase one. You may feel some excess gas as you are incorporating so much more fiber in your diet than you were before. That is normal and you will eventually adjust. If you find it bothersome, scale back on the beans and substitute another dish. The meal plan will ease up a little bit in phase two, allowing you some more variation, but you will continue to see health benefits and improvements as you make your way through phase one.

SNACKS TO ENJOY:

- Handful of almonds
- ½ cup of fresh raspberries
- ½ cup of fresh blueberries
- Yogurt with pineapple chunks
- Jicama slices
- Hardboiled egg with salt and pepper

- ½ cup Kimchi with Sesame Seeds (page 214), or store-bought
- Mandarin orange and ½ cup yogurt
- Celery topped with Roasted Red Pepper Hummus (page 182)
- Red and green pepper strips with Beet Dip (page 180)

Week Three Shopping List

CANNED / BOTTLED / PACKAGED FOODS

Black beans, low-sodium
(2 (15-ounce) cans)
Chickpeas, low-sodium
(2 [15-ounce] cans)
Chipotle chiles in adobo sauce
(1 [12-ounce] can)
Fermented vegetables
(1 [16-ounce] jar, or
make them yourself—
see chapter 12)
Pineapple, in its own juices
(1 [8-ounce] can)
Shirataki noodles (1 [7-ounce]
package)
Tomatoes, whole, fire-roasted
(4 [15-ounce] cans)
Tomatoes, whole, fire-roasted
(1 [28-ounce] can)
Tuna, packed in water
(1 [6-ounce] can)
Vegetable broth, low-sodium
(2 [32-ounce] containers)

DAIRY AND EGGS

Kefir, plain, (1 cup, or make
your own—see page 211)
Large eggs (half dozen)
Parmesan cheese, shredded
(4 ounces)
Yogurt, unsweetened, plain
(1 quart)

PANTRY STAPLES

Almonds, raw
Almonds, sliced
Basil, dried
Black pepper
Cashews, raw
Cayenne pepper, ground
Chia seeds, whole
Cinnamon, ground
Coriander, ground
Cumin, ground
Dates, whole, pitted
Flaxseed, ground
Flaxseed, whole
Garlic powder
Lentils, brown
Lentils, French green
Mustard, whole-grain
Nonstick cooking spray
Oats, rolled, gluten-free
Oats, steel cut, gluten-free
Oil, extra-virgin olive
Oil, sesame
Onion powder
Oregano, dried
Paprika, smoked
Raisins, golden
Red pepper flakes
Salt
Tamari
Thyme, dried
Turmeric, ground
Vanilla extract
Vinegar, rice
Vinegar, white
Walnuts, pieces

MEAT AND SEAFOOD

Cod fillets (1 pound)
Shrimp, large (1 pound)

PRODUCE

Banana (1)
Basil, fresh (1 bunch)
Bell pepper, green (1)
Bell pepper, red (1)
Blueberries (1 pint)
Broccoli (8 ounces)
Carrots (5)
Celery (1 bunch)
Chard (1 bunch)
Cilantro, fresh (1 bunch)
Garlic, fresh (2 heads)
Ginger, fresh (1 knob)
Grapes (8 ounces)
Kale (4 bunches)
Lemons (3)
Limes (3)
Mint, fresh (1 bunch)
Mushrooms, cremini (4 ounces)
Onions, yellow (5)
Parsley, fresh (1 bunch)
Raspberries (1 pint)
Scallions (2 bunches)
Spaghetti squash (1)
Tomatoes (3)

OTHER

Almond milk, plain,
unsweetened (half gallon)
Tofu, soft (12 ounces)
Tofu, firm (12 ounces)
White cooking wine, dry
(1 [300-millileter] bottle)

Week Three Meal Plan

	BREAKFAST	LUNCH	DINNER
MONDAY	Oat and Nut Muesli with Raspberries (page 86) and almond milk	Chickpea, Tomato, and Kale Soup (page 103) and ¼ cup fermented vegetables	Shrimp Scampi and Greens (page 152)
TUESDAY	Vanilla Chia Seed Pudding with Strawberries and Almonds (page 91)	Tuna Salad Lettuce Wraps (page 146)	Moroccan Date and Carrot Lentil Salad (page 129) and ¼ cup fermented vegetables
WEDNESDAY	Overnight Oatmeal with Fruit and Nuts (page 88)	Simple Lentil Soup (page 99) and Simple Green Side Salad (page 107)	Black Bean and Quinoa Bowl (page 131)
THURSDAY	Blueberry Banana Protein Burst (page 73)	Leftover Moroccan Date and Carrot Lentil Salad	Shirataki, Vegetable, and Tofu Stir-Fry (page 138)
FRIDAY	Oat and Nut Muesli with Raspberries (page 86)	Leftover Black Bean and Quinoa Bowl	Blackened Cod with Pineapple Salsa (page 153) and Cauliflower Rice (page 188)
SATURDAY	Poached Eggs on a Bed of Kale Pesto and Tomatoes (page 80)	Leftover Shirataki, Vegetable, and Tofu Stir-Fry	Black Bean Chili (page 102) and ¼ cup fermented vegetables
SUNDAY	Probiotic Cinnamon Steel Cut Oats (page 87) with ½ cup fruit	Egg and Beet Spinach Salad (page 113) and leftover Cauliflower Rice	Marinara Spaghetti Squash Noodles (page 122) and ¼ cup fermented vegetables

GET AHEAD

Sunday: Make the Oat and Nut Muesli with Raspberries (page 86), which is an energizing ready-to-go breakfast, to enjoy throughout the week. Cook up a batch each of Chickpea, Tomato, and Kale Soup (page 103) and Simple Lentil Soup (page 99). Prepare the Tuna Salad Lettuce Wraps (page 146) through step 2 for lunch on Tuesday.

Tuesday: Prepare the Overnight Oatmeal with Fruit and Nuts (page 88).

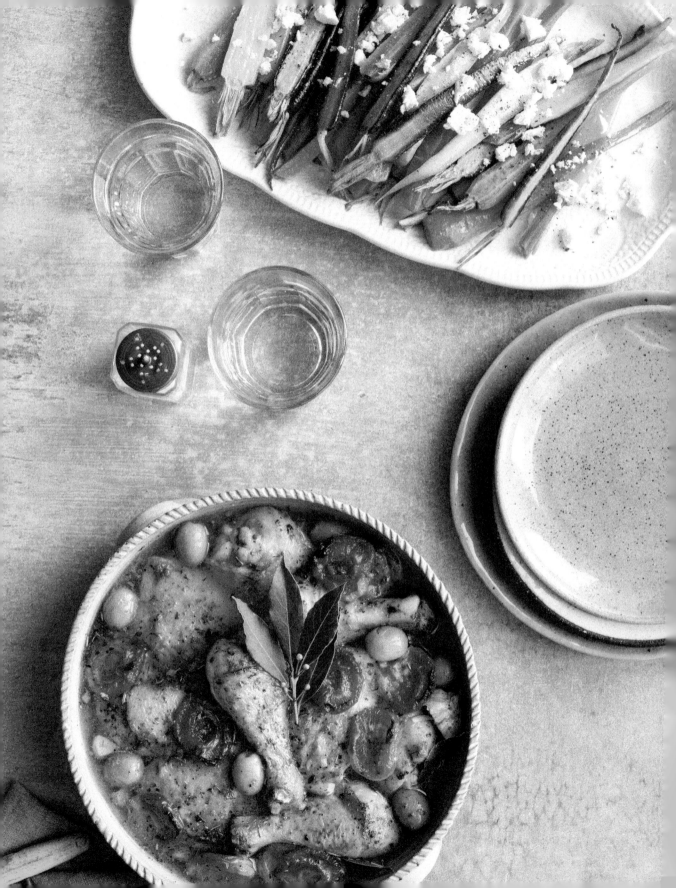

Phase Two Meal Plan
Sustain

You did it! Congratulations on making it to phase two of the microbiome meal plan. Give yourself a hug for getting this far, and know that your microbes are thanking you. Things are going to ease up a little bit now, as you will be adding back in small amounts of meat and some sweetness (in the form of maple syrup or honey). You will be maintaining your intake of probiotic foods and high-fiber carbohydrates, which by now your gut probably loves.

Week Four

One of the big changes in phase two is the reintroduction of some meat, including beef, pork, and chicken. Of course, if you don't want to add it back in, you can easily substitute one of the vegetarian or fish recipes; the plan is meant to be manageable and adjustable. As always, check in with yourself to see how you feel. Does adding meat back into your diet make a difference? Did you miss it or not crave it as much as you thought? You have a tempting list of meals this week . . . so go for it!

SNACKS TO ENJOY:

- Handful of almonds
- Handful of grapes
- ½ cup of fresh blueberries
- Yogurt with mango chunks
- Radishes dipped in Asparagus Hummus (page 181)
- ½ cup diced cantaloupe
- Piece of hard cheese and a handful of walnuts
- Handful of Cinnamon Almonds (page 183)
- ½ cup Kimchi with Sesame Seeds (page 214), or store-bought
- Fermented vegetables

Week Four Shopping List

CANNED / BOTTLED / PACKAGED FOODS

Black beans, low-sodium
  (2 [15-ounce] cans)
Beef broth, low-sodium
  (1 [32-ounce] package)
Chicken broth, low-sodium
  (1 [32-ounce] package)
Fermented vegetables
  (1 [16-ounce] jar, or
  make them yourself—
  see chapter 12)
Kalamata olives, pitted
  (1 [6-ounce] jar)
Salmon, boneless, skinless
  (1 [6-ounce] can)
Vegetable broth, low-sodium
  (1 [16-ounce] container)

DAIRY AND EGGS

Blue cheese, crumbled
  (4 ounces)
Kefir, plain (1 quart, or make
  your own—see page 211)
Large eggs (1 dozen)
Parmesan cheese, shredded
  (2 ounces)
Yogurt, unsweetened, plain
  (1 quart)

PANTRY STAPLES

Almond butter
Baking soda
Black pepper
Cinnamon, ground
Cocoa powder, unsweetened
Cumin, ground
Flaxseed, ground
Garlic powder
Ginger powder
Honey
Lentils, French green
Mayonnaise
Mustard, Dijon
Nonstick cooking spray
Oats, rolled, gluten-free
Oats, steel cut, gluten-free
Oil, canola
Oil, extra-virgin olive
Oil, sesame
Oregano, dried
Paprika, smoked
Peanut butter
Peanuts, raw
Raisins, golden
Red pepper flakes
Rice, brown
Salt
Sesame seeds, whole
Tamari
Turmeric
Vanilla extract
Vinegar, rice
Vinegar, red wine
Vinegar, white
Walnuts, pieces

MEAT AND SEAFOOD

Beef, boneless sirloin (1 pound)
Chicken, boneless, skinless
  breasts (2 pounds)
Cod fillets (1 pound)

PRODUCE

Avocado (2)
Banana (3)
Beets (4)
Blueberries (1 pint)
Carrots (1 pound)
Cauliflower (1 head)
Celery (1 bunch)
Cilantro, fresh (1 bunch)
Cucumber (1)
Eggplant, medium (2)
Garlic, fresh (1 head)
Ginger, fresh (1 knob)
Grapes (8 ounces)
Kale (2 bunches)
Jalapeño pepper (1)
Lemons (4)
Lettuce, red or green leaf
  (3 heads)
Lettuce, romaine (2 heads)
Lime (1)
Mint, fresh (1 bunch)
Onions, yellow (5)
Oranges, mandarin (3)
Parsley, fresh (1 bunch)
Parsnip (1)
Potatoes, russet (3)
Scallions (3 bunches)
Tomatoes, medium (5)
Turnip (1)
Zucchini (1)

OTHER

Almond milk, plain,
  unsweetened (half gallon)

Week Four Meal Plan

	BREAKFAST	LUNCH	DINNER
MONDAY	Oat, Walnut, and Golden Raisin Granola (page 85) with yogurt	Italian Lentil Salad (page 127)	Chinese Chicken Lettuce Wraps (page 163) and Simple Green Side Salad (page 107)
TUESDAY	Chocolate, Peanut Butter, and Zucchini Muffins (page 84) with yogurt	Chicken Salad on a Bed of Greens (page 162)	Beet Yogurt Soup (page 95) and Asian Kale Salad with Sesame-Ginger Dressing (page 108)
WEDNESDAY	Oat, Walnut, and Golden Raisin Granola (page 85) with nondairy milk and ½ cup blueberries	Salmon Salad Lettuce Wraps (page 145) and ¼ cup fermented vegetables	Kung Pao Chickpeas (page 136) with Cauliflower Rice (page 188)
THURSDAY	Probiotic Cinnamon Steel Cut Oats (page 87)	Leftover Chicken Salad on a Bed of Greens and ¼ cup fermented vegetables	Brown Rice–Stuffed Eggplant (page 126)
FRIDAY	Chocolate Almond Smoothie (page 71)	Leftover Beet Yogurt Soup, leftover Asian Kale Salad with Sesame-Ginger Dressing and ¼ cup fermented vegetables	Chicken and Brown Rice Soup (page 105)
SATURDAY	Brown Rice and Egg Breakfast Bowl with Kimchi (page 81)	Leftover Brown Rice–Stuffed Eggplant	Beef and Root Vegetable Stew (page 106) and Sweet and Savory Orange Walnut Salad (page 111)
SUNDAY	Poached Eggs on a Bed of Kale Pesto and Tomatoes (page 80)	Black Bean Burrito Bowl (page 132) and ¼ cup fermented vegetables	Corn and Whitefish Chowder (page 104)

GET AHEAD

Sunday: Make the Oat, Walnut, and Golden Raisin Granola (page 85) for a satisfying, tasty start to the week. Also make the Simple Baked Chicken Breasts (page 159) in preparation for Monday's dinner and Tuesday's lunch. Prepare the Italian Lentil Salad (page 127).

Monday: Prepare the Chicken Salad on a Bed of Greens (page 162) through step 2 for Tuesday.

Week Five

You are getting close to the finish line. You have some more awesome recipes to try this week to keep you motivated. Some of these recipes may sound exotic, but as always they include ingredients that you can find in your grocery store, and they won't keep you slaving over the stove. As in the other weeks, leftovers are incorporated so that you won't be cooking three meals a day even though you will be eating three homemade meals a day. How are you feeling? You may notice that your clothes are fitting more comfortably and that your mood has improved. As you embark on this fifth week of the microbiome diet, you already have a whole month behind you of probiotic-powered, high-fiber, delicious meals. You should feel really good about yourself for what you have achieved so far (and your gut should be feeling really good too!).

SNACKS TO ENJOY:

- ½ cup strawberries, raspberries, or blueberries
- ½ Raspberry Smoothie (page 75)
- Yogurt and 1 mandarin orange
- Kale or Sunchoke Chips (page 185)
- Apple slices with nut butter
- Handful of Fruit and Nut Trail Mix (page 187)
- Dried bananas
- Hardboiled egg with salt and pepper
- Handful of grapes
- 1 kiwi fruit

Week Five Shopping List

CANNED / BOTTLED / PACKAGED FOODS

Butter beans,
    (2 [15-ounce] cans)
Chicken broth, low-sodium
    (1 [16-ounce] container)
Chickpeas, low-sodium
    (1 [15-ounce] can)
Fermented vegetables
    (1 [16-ounce] jar, or
    make them yourself—
    see chapter 12)
Tomatoes, diced
    (1 [15-ounce] can)
Tomatoes, whole
    (2 [28-ounce] cans)
Vegetable broth, low-sodium
    (2 [32-ounce] containers)

DAIRY AND EGGS

Feta cheese, crumbled
    (8 ounces)
Goat cheese, crumbled
    (4 ounces)
Kefir, plain (1 quart, or make
    your own—see page 211)
Large eggs (half dozen)
Yogurt, unsweetened, plain
    (1 quart)

FROZEN FOODS

Raspberries (16 ounces)

PANTRY STAPLES

Almonds, sliced
Almonds, whole
Almond flour
Black pepper
Buckwheat groats
Cashews, whole
Chia seeds, whole
Cinnamon, ground
Coconut, dried, unsweetened

Coriander, ground
Cumin, ground
Flaxseed, ground
Flaxseed, whole
Garlic powder
Ginger powder
Honey
Lentils, brown or French green
Mustard, Dijon
Nonstick cooking spray
Oats, rolled, gluten-free
Oats, steel cut, gluten-free
Oil, canola
Oil, extra-virgin olive
Paprika, smoked
Pecan, halves
Quinoa
Raisins, golden
Red pepper flakes
Salt
Sesame seeds, whole
Thyme, dried
Turmeric, ground
Vanilla extract
Vinegar, balsamic
Vinegar, red wine
Vinegar, white wine
Walnuts, pieces

MEAT AND SEAFOOD

Chicken, bone-in breasts (2)
Chicken, boneless skinless
    breasts (2)
Chicken, leg quarters (4)
Salmon fillets (1 pound)

PRODUCE

Arugula (5 ounces)
Avocado (1)
Banana (1)
Basil, fresh (1 bunch)
Beets (2)
Bell pepper, green (1)
Bell pepper, red (1)
Blueberries (1 pint)
Brussels sprouts (1 pound)
Carrots (6)
Cauliflower (2 heads)
Celery (1 bunch)
Cilantro, fresh (1 cup)
Cucumber (1)
Fennel (1 bulb)
Garlic, fresh (2 heads)
Ginger, fresh (1 knob)
Kohlrabi (1 bulb)
Lemons (5)
Lettuce, red or green leaf
    (3 heads)
Lettuce, romaine (2 heads)
Mushrooms, cremini (6 ounces)
Onions, yellow (4)
Parsley, fresh (1 bunch)
Pear (1)
Pomegranate (1)
Radishes (1 bunch)
Raspberries (1 pint)
Rosemary, fresh (2 sprigs)
Scallions (8)
Shallots (5)
Swiss chard (1 bunch)
Sweet potato (9 ounces)
Strawberries (1 pint)
Tomatoes (2)
Turnips (1 pound)

OTHER

Almond milk, plain,
    unsweetened (half gallon)
Tofu, firm (12 ounces)
Tofu, soft (12 ounces)

Week Five Meal Plan

	BREAKFAST	LUNCH	DINNER
MONDAY	Yogurt Parfait (page 89) with blueberries	Goat Cheese and Lentil Salad (page 128)	Cauliflower Rice Chicken Biriyani (page 169)
TUESDAY	Raspberry Smoothie (page 75)	Arugula and Walnut Quinoa Bowl (page 121)	Mushroom Tofu Burgers (page 140), Gazpacho Salad (page 110), and ¼ cup fermented vegetables
WEDNESDAY	Oat and Nut Muesli with Raspberries (page 86) and almond milk	Leftover Goat Cheese and Lentil Salad with leftover Gazpacho Salad	Chicken and Root Vegetable Roast (page 167) and ¼ cup fermented vegetables
THURSDAY	Blueberry Banana Protein Burst (page 73)	Leftover Cauliflower Rice Chicken Biriyani	Creamy Tomato Soup (page 98), Simple Green Side Salad (page 107), and ¼ cup fermented vegetables
FRIDAY	Vanilla Chia Seed Pudding with Strawberries and Almonds (page 91)	Leftover Mushroom Tofu Burgers and Simple Green Side Salad (page 107)	One-Pan Salmon, Sweet Potato, and Brussels Sprouts Bake (page 155)
SATURDAY	Poached egg with leftover Cauliflower Rice	Simple Lentil Soup (page 99), Fragrant Fennel and Kohlrabi Salad (page 109), and ¼ cup fermented vegetables	Chicken, Tomatoes, and White Bean Bake (page 170)
SUNDAY	Probiotic Cinnamon Steel Cut Oats (page 87)	Winter Pear, Beet, and Pomegranate Salad (page 112)	Chickpea and Avocado Buckwheat Tabbouleh (page 134) and Simple Green Side Salad (page 107)

GET AHEAD

Sunday: Make the Oat and Nut Muesli with Raspberries (page 86) for breakfast on Wednesday. Prepare the Goat Cheese and Lentil Salad (page 128) through step 2, and mix up the dressing.

Monday: Prep the Arugula and Walnut Quinoa Bowl (page 121).

Thursday: Prep the Vanilla Chia Seed Pudding with Strawberries and Almonds (page 91) for Friday's breakfast, and prep the Chicken, Apricot, and Olive Bake (page 168), which you'll be enjoying for Friday's dinner.

Week Six

You have made it to the last week of the microbiome diet! Treat yourself with some Chocolate, Peanut Butter, and Zucchini Muffins (page 84). How are you feeling? You are about to complete your six-week journey to revamp and optimize your gut microbiome, and you're likely looking and feeling your very best. You've probably lost some weight too. The hope is that you now love this new way of eating and that it will become a part of your lifestyle. You can continue to utilize these recipes well beyond this six-week plan. Bookmark your favorite recipes so that you can come back and reference them at any time.

SNACKS TO ENJOY:

- ¼ cup Kimchi with Sesame Seeds (page 214) mixed with 2 tablespoons of cooked quinoa
- ½ cup grapes
- Kohlrabi or jicama sticks
- Red and green bell pepper sticks
- Celery sticks with peanut butter
- Cauliflower florets dipped in hummus
- ½ cup Sauerkraut (page 212)
- ½ cup Fermented Cauliflower, Carrots, and Red Onions (page 215)
- Yogurt with fresh berries
- ½ cup diced melon

Week Six Shopping List

CANNED / BOTTLED / PACKAGED FOODS

Chickpeas, low-sodium
 (3 [15-ounce] cans)
Kalamata olives, pitted
 (1 [9-ounce] jar)
Kimchi (1 [16-ounce] jar,
 or make it yourself—see
 Kimchi with Sesame Seeds
 [page 214])
Fermented vegetables
 (1 [16-ounce] jar, or
 make them yourself—
 see chapter 12)
Tomato paste (1 [5-ounce] can)
Tomatoes, whole
 (1 [15-ounce] can)
Tomatoes, whole
 (1 [28-ounce] can)
Vegetable broth, low-sodium
 (1 [32-ounce] container)

DAIRY AND EGGS

Blue cheese, crumbled
 (4 ounces)
Feta cheese, crumbled
 (8 ounces)
Goat cheese, crumbled
 (4 ounces)
Kefir, plain (1 quart, or make it
 yourself—see page 211)
Large eggs (1 dozen)
Mozzarella cheese, shredded
 (4 ounces)
Parmesan cheese, shredded
 (4 ounces)
Yogurt, unsweetened, plain
 (1 quart)

FROZEN FOODS

Blackberries (16 ounces)
Mangos (16 ounces)

PANTRY STAPLES

Almonds, sliced
Baking soda
Black pepper
Chia seeds, whole
Cocoa powder, unsweetened
Flaxseed, ground
Honey
Lentils, French green
Millet
Mustard, Dijon
Mustard, whole-grain
Nonstick cooking spray
Oats, rolled, gluten-free
Oil, canola
Oil, sesame
Oil, extra-virgin olive
Peanut butter, natural
Peanuts, unsalted
Red pepper flakes, crushed
Salt
Tamari
Turmeric, ground
Vanilla extract
Vinegar, red wine
Vinegar, rice
Walnuts, pieces

MEAT AND SEAFOOD

Beef, flank steak (2 pounds)
Beef, ground, lean (8 ounces)
Chicken, boneless, skinless
 breasts (8 ounces)

PRODUCE

Avocado (1)
Bananas (2)
Basil, fresh (2 bunches)
Bell peppers, green (3)
Bell peppers, red (6)
Blueberries (2 pints)
Broccoli, florets (50 ounces)
Cabbage, red (1 head)
Cantaloupe (1)
Carrots (1)
Cauliflower (3 heads)
Celery (1 bunch)
Garlic, fresh (1 head)
Ginger, fresh (1 knob)
Grapes (8 ounces)
Kiwi fruit (1)
Lemons (2)
Lettuce, red or green leaf
 (3 heads)
Mushrooms, cremini (4 ounces)
Onions, yellow (3)
Onion, red (1)
Oranges, mandarin (3)
Salad greens (1 [15-ounce]
 package)
Scallions (8)
Spinach, baby (12 ounces)
Raspberries (1 pint)
Tomatoes (3)
Zucchini, medium (9)

OTHER

Almond milk, plain,
 unsweetened (1 quart)
Rice cooking wine or sake
 (1 [300-millileter] bottle)
Tofu, firm (1 [12-ounce]
 package)

Week Six Meal Plan

	BREAKFAST	LUNCH	DINNER
MONDAY	Chocolate, Peanut Butter, and Zucchini Muffins (page 84) with ½ cup fruit	Tofu and Lentil Salad (page 114)	Mediterranean Millet-Stuffed Peppers (page 124) and ¼ cup fermented vegetables
TUESDAY	Blueberry Ginger Smoothie (page 72)	Creamy Tomato Soup (page 98) and Broccoli and Olive Salad (page 116)	Pesto Zucchini Noodles with Tomatoes (page 123) and ¼ cup fermented vegetables
WEDNESDAY	Tropical Turmeric Kefir Smoothie (page 74)	Tuna Salad Lettuce Wraps (page 146)	Chicken and Broccoli Stir-Fry (page 166) and Cauliflower Rice (page 188)
THURSDAY	Overnight Oatmeal with Fruit and Nuts (page 88)	Leftover Mediterranean Millet-Stuffed Peppers and ¼ cup fermented vegetables	Kung Pao Chickpeas (page 136) and leftover Cauliflower Rice
FRIDAY	Chia Yogurt Melon Bowl (page 90)	Sweet and Savory Orange Walnut Salad (page 111)	Italian Lentil Salad (page 127)
SATURDAY	Brown Rice and Egg Breakfast Bowl with Kimchi (page 81)	Chicken and Quinoa Salad Bowl (page 161)	Slow Cooker Korean Beef Tacos with Red Slaw (page 174)
SUNDAY	Make-Ahead Egg and Vegetable Cups (page 76)	Leftover Italian Lentil Salad	Beef and Cauliflower Bake (page 172) and ¼ cup fermented vegetables

GET AHEAD

Sunday: Make the Chocolate Peanut Butter, and Zucchini Muffins (page 84) and look forward to Monday's breakfast treat. Prepare the Tofu and Lentil Salad (page 114) through step 3. Cook up a batch of Creamy Tomato Soup (page 98). Prepare the Broccoli and Olive Salad (page 116).

Wednesday: Prep your Overnight Oatmeal with Fruit and Nuts (page 88) for breakfast on Thursday.

Thursday: Prep the Chia Yogurt Melon Bowl (page 90) and refrigerate overnight. Make the Italian Lentil Salad (page 127).

Make the Plan a Lifestyle

Supporting your microbiome means making changes that go beyond a six-week meal plan and become a way of life. The recipes in this book provide you with countless possibilities to continue eating in a way that will support your microbiome, your weight goals, and your overall health, even after you're finished with the meal plan. Now, even though you have more than enough recipes to keep you going, most of you are not going to be able to eat every single meal at home. Do what you can, and if you have to attend an event where you cannot bring your own dish, try to stick to the principles while you are dining out: Focus on high-fiber grains, vegetables, and fermented foods when possible. Even if you do manage to prepare all your meals, there will be some days you just feel like you need a brownie. Before giving in to the temptation, think about how you will feel after eating it—or any other sugary or processed food. Will it be worth it? Ideally, you will stick to this program completely for six weeks and then incorporate these types of meals into your lifestyle. If you can follow the microbiome diet principles more than 90 percent of the time, you're doing really well.

In addition to diet, here are some lifestyle changes that can help you maintain a healthy weight and feel great while you're at it.

Get rested: Your body functions best when you get sufficient sleep, and that counts for your microbes too. There is even research that shows that disruptions to your sleep schedule can affect the microbial diversity of your gut, so you want to make sure that you and your microbes get enough high-quality rest.

Get moving: Exercising, even something as simple as getting out of your chair and taking a walk for 20 minutes, can be beneficial to your digestive health. First of all, it gets your system moving. When you move, your digestive system moves too. Plus—you guessed it—there is emerging research that looks at exercise and, yes, it affects your microbiome in a good way.

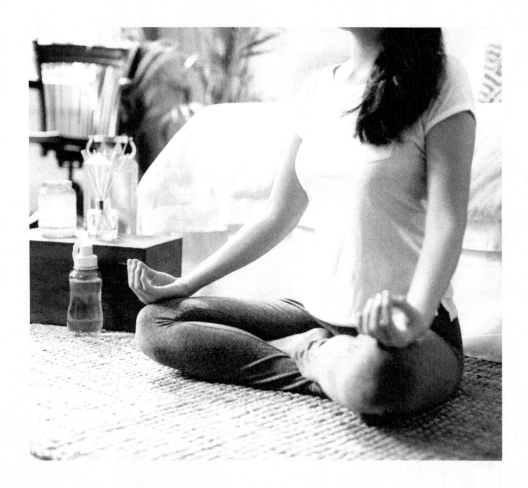

Get relaxed: Reducing stress is something that will make you and your microbes feel better. Stress has significant adverse consequences on your gut, and will counteract all the effort that you are making in your diet. This is why the diet plan is designed to be as stress-free as possible! So treat yourself to some self-care and relaxation—maybe it's a phone call with a friend, a walk in the park, or a warm bubble bath. Whatever works for you, make sure that you do something for yourself every single day.

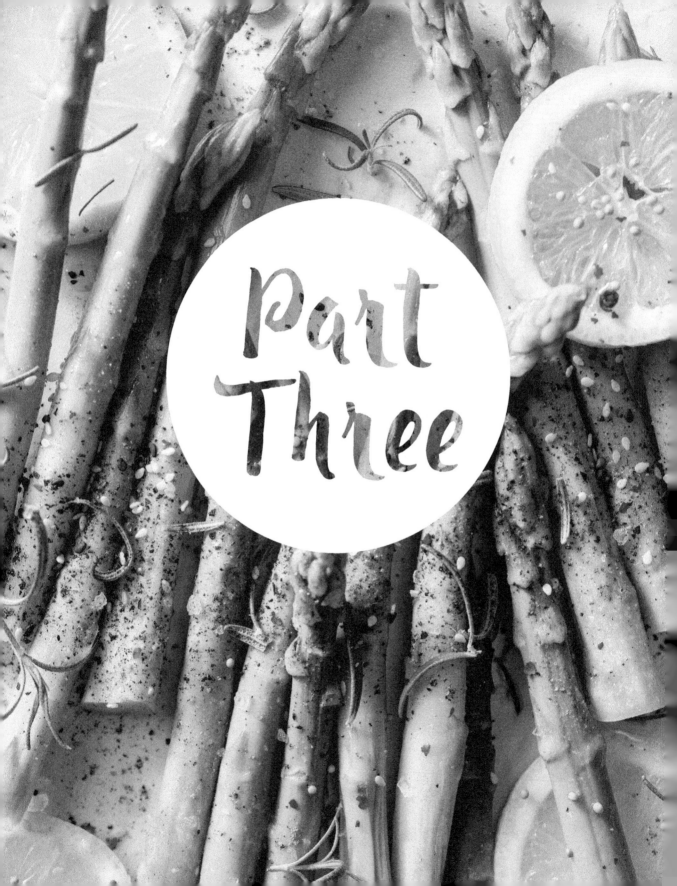

Part
Three

The Recipes

Now we get to the fun stuff. Here you will find more than 120 recipes to transform your microbiome into a happy, healthy, properly functioning community of microbes. And when your microbiome is happy, your body will be happy. Use the meal plans provided in part two, or mix and match the recipes according to your preferences, taking into account which phase you are in (each recipe will be marked phase one or two). All the recipes are gluten-free. Each recipe also has labels to help you if you're looking for something dairy-free, grain-free, nut-free, vegan, or "under 30 minutes."

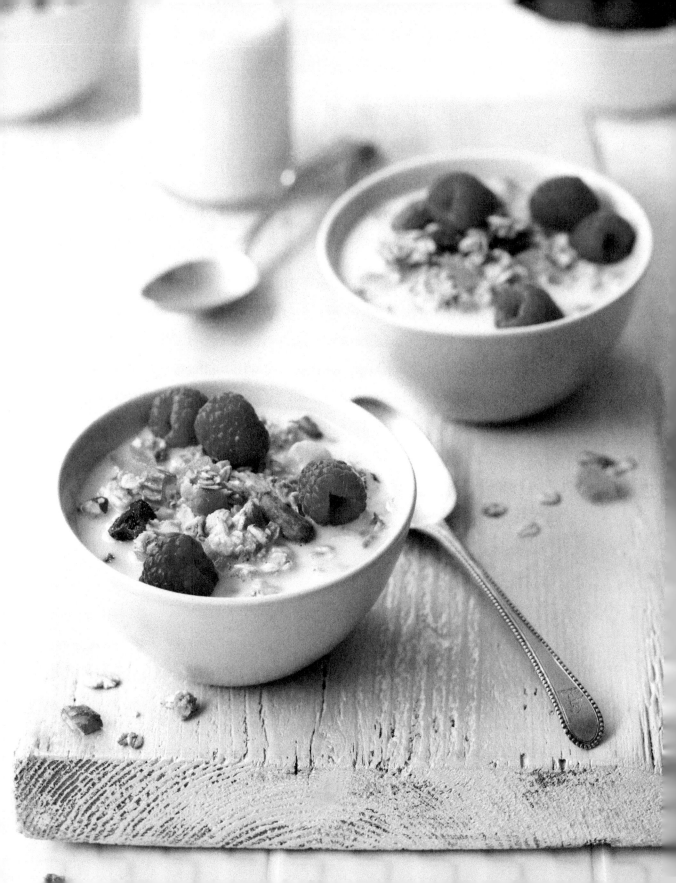

Breakfast and Smoothies

Breakfast is said to be the most important meal of the day. It is even *more* important when changing your eating habits because it ensures that hunger doesn't lead to poor food choices. These meals are designed to fill you up and give you the energy you need to power through your day. Mix and match these tasty meals throughout the week for a balanced and sensible approach to your first meal of the day.

Chocolate Almond Smoothie

DAIRY-FREE | GRAIN-FREE | VEGAN | UNDER 30 MINUTES

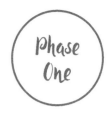

Phase One

Chocolate is an unlikely suspect to find in a breakfast recipe in a diet book. But just because the sumptuous cocoa bean, from which chocolate is derived, is so often paired with all varieties of sugar, it doesn't mean chocolate has to be shunned. Mix the unsweetened powder with banana and almond and you have a healthy, diet-worthy drink that will keep you energized throughout the morning. **SERVES 1**

Place all the ingredients in a blender and process until smooth. Serve.

TIP Look for unsweetened cocoa powder in the baking section of your grocery store. Either regular unsweetened cocoa powder or Dutch process cocoa powder are acceptable choices for this recipe.

Per Serving: Calories: 351; Protein: 11g; Cholesterol: 0mg; Sodium: 252mg; Total Carbohydrates: 37g; Fiber: 11g; Total Fat: 23g; Saturated Fat: 2g

PREP TIME: 5 MINUTES

1 cup unsweetened plain almond milk

2 tablespoons almond butter

2 tablespoons unsweetened cocoa powder

1 banana

4 or 5 ice cubes

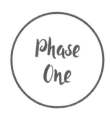

PREP TIME: 5 MINUTES

½ cup unsweetened
almond milk

1 cup blueberries

2 tablespoons chia seeds

½ cup unsweetened
plain yogurt

1 (2-inch) piece fresh
ginger, minced

4 or 5 ice cubes

Blueberry Ginger Smoothie

GRAIN-FREE | NUT-FREE | UNDER 30 MINUTES

Ginger adds a complex spiciness to anything it touches.
Ginger is also good for you—it stimulates digestion and
improves circulation, making it a perfect ingredient
to start your day. Combined with blueberries for a
mild sweetness, chia seeds for a dose of omega-3 fatty
acids, and yogurt for probiotics and protein, this is a
nutrient-dense breakfast smoothie with a zip. **SERVES 1**

Place all the ingredients in a blender and process until
smooth. Serve.

Per Serving: Calories: 431; Protein: 16g; Cholesterol: 11mg; Sodium: 202mg;
Total Carbohydrates: 41g; Fiber: 17g; Total Fat: 26g; Saturated Fat: 6g

Blueberry Banana Protein Burst

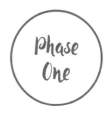

Phase One

DAIRY-FREE | GRAIN-FREE | VEGAN | UNDER 30 MINUTES

PREP TIME: 5 MINUTES

Tofu is often overlooked for this purpose, but is perfect to use in a smoothie. It is a great dairy-free protein source that creates a rich creaminess and adds little actual flavor, allowing it to take on the taste of whatever you blend it with. This smoothie is sweetened with blueberries and a banana, and uses half of a standard block of tofu, enabling you to save some for another meal later in the week. **SERVES 1**

Place all the ingredients in a blender and process until smooth. Serve.

6 ounces soft tofu

½ cup unsweetened plain almond milk

¼ cup blueberries

1 banana

½ teaspoon ground cinnamon

4 or 5 ice cubes

MAKE AHEAD All smoothies can be made ahead to save time; however, they will need to be remixed in the morning for the best consistency. To make things simple, you can prep all the ingredients in the blender and refrigerate it overnight. In the morning, simply process and serve for a tasty meal in a snap.

Per Serving: Calories: 254; Protein: 14g; Cholesterol: 0mg; Sodium: 195mg; Total Carbohydrates: 33g; Fiber: 5g; Total Fat: 10g; Saturated Fat: 1g

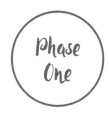

Phase
One

PREP TIME: 5 MINUTES

1 cup Kefir (page 211) or
  store-bought
½ cup frozen
  mango chunks
½ cup frozen blackberries
½ banana
1 teaspoon ground turmeric

Tropical Turmeric Kefir Smoothie

GRAIN-FREE | NUT-FREE | UNDER 30 MINUTES

This smoothie uses kefir for its creamy base. Slightly different in taste from yogurt, kefir is a cultured dairy product that can be widely enjoyed on the microbiome diet. Here it is combined with the anti-inflammatory spice turmeric to create a slightly sweet, tropical smoothie with a bite. SERVES 1

Place all the ingredients in a blender and process until smooth. Serve.

DID YOU KNOW? Curcumin, the yellow pigment that gives turmeric its color, accounts for its status as one of the best sources of beta-carotene. Although tumeric is a powerful antioxidant and is also antibacterial, it is perhaps best known for its anti-inflammatory properties. It is commonly used in Indian cooking and makes its way into many chili powders and spice blends.

Per Serving: Calories: 310; Protein: 11g; Cholesterol: 35mg; Sodium: 125mg; Total Carbohydrates: 48g; Fiber: 7g; Total Fat: 10g; Saturated Fat: 5g

Raspberry Smoothie

GRAIN-FREE | NUT-FREE | UNDER 30 MINUTES

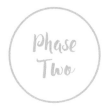

This raspberry smoothie tastes like summer in a glass. It is a no-nonsense, three-ingredient treat that makes a light meal or post-workout snack. Because it uses honey to cut the tart kefir flavor, you will have to wait until phase two to enjoy this one. **SERVES 1**

Place all the ingredients in a blender and process until smooth. Serve.

Per Serving: Calories: 248; Protein: 10g; Cholesterol: 35mg; Sodium: 124mg; Total Carbohydrates: 33g; Fiber: 9g; Total Fat: 10g; Saturated Fat: 5g

PREP TIME: 5 MINUTES

1 cup frozen raspberries

1 cup Kefir (page 211) or store-bought

1 teaspoon honey

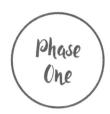

Phase One

PREP TIME: 10 MINUTES
COOK TIME: 25 MINUTES

Nonstick cooking spray

1 tablespoon extra-virgin olive oil

1 cup finely diced red bell pepper

1 cup finely diced green bell pepper

1 cup finely diced yellow onion

1 cup finely chopped cremini mushrooms

2 cups packed roughly chopped baby spinach leaves

1 garlic clove, chopped

½ teaspoon salt

¼ teaspoon freshly ground black pepper

6 eggs

½ cup shredded Parmesan cheese

Make-Ahead Egg *and* Vegetable Cups

GRAIN-FREE | NUT-FREE

Getting enough protein in the morning is imperative in order to have plenty of energy to keep you going until lunch. These quick egg cups are simple to throw together in advance. Whip up a batch on a lazy weekend day to make your weekday mornings quick, easy, and delicious. SERVES 6

1. Preheat the oven to 350°F.

2. Lightly spray the cups of a muffin tin with cooking spray.

3. In a large skillet, heat the oil over medium-high heat. Add the red and green peppers and the onion to the skillet and cook for 5 to 7 minutes, until softened.

4. Add the mushrooms, spinach, and garlic and stir constantly until the spinach just wilts. Season with the salt and pepper. Remove the skillet from the heat.

5. In a large mixing bowl, whisk the eggs lightly. Stir in the cheese and the cooked vegetables.

6. Pour the mixture evenly into the muffin tin, filling all 12 cups.

7. Bake for 15 minutes, until the egg has set and the tops are firm.

8. Cool for 5 minutes, remove them from the muffin tin, and serve. Refrigerate any leftovers in an airtight container for up to 4 days.

MAKE AHEAD You can freeze these and stock them up for later. To do so, store them in the freezer in an airtight container for up to 1 month. When ready to eat, heat them in the microwave for 1 to 2 minutes.

Per Serving: Calories: 159; Protein: 11g; Cholesterol: 213mg; Sodium: 398mg; Total Carbohydrates: 7g; Fiber: 2g; Total Fat: 10g; Saturated Fat: 3g

Make-Ahead Tofu *and* Vegetable Frittatas

DAIRY-FREE | GRAIN-FREE | NUT-FREE | VEGAN

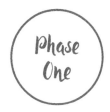

Phase One

Make these mini frittatas ahead and have a quick breakfast or lunch ready when you need it. Loaded with vegetables, these simple finger foods are packed with protein to keep you energized. Don't overlook their ability to transform lunchtime as well—paired with a salad, they are filling and ensure you get your daily dose of veggies. **SERVES 6**

PREP TIME: 10 MINUTES
COOK TIME: 30 MINUTES

Nonstick cooking spray

1 (12-ounce) package extra-firm tofu

1 tablespoon nutritional yeast

2 tablespoons tamari

1 teaspoon extra-virgin olive oil

1 small potato, finely diced

1 red bell pepper, finely diced

½ cup diced yellow onion

2 cups thinly sliced spinach leaves

¼ cup chopped fresh basil leaves

2 garlic cloves, minced

1. Preheat the oven to 350°F.

2. Lightly spray the cups of a muffin tin with cooking spray.

3. In a blender, combine the tofu, nutritional yeast, and tamari. Process until smooth and set aside.

4. In a large skillet, heat the oil over medium-high heat. Add the potato to the skillet and cook for 5 minutes, until it starts to brown. Add the bell pepper and onion to the skillet and cook for 5 to 7 minutes, until softened.

5. Add the spinach, basil, and garlic to the skillet and stir constantly until the spinach just wilts.

6. Add the tofu mixture to the vegetables and stir to combine.

7. Scoop the mixture evenly into the muffin tin, filling all 12 cups. Bake for 15 to 20 minutes, until the tops have slightly browned and the frittatas are firm.

INGREDIENT TIP Nutritional yeast is also commonly called brewer's yeast. It is extremely rich in B vitamins and has a distinct nutty taste. Look for it at health food stores, bulk-food sections, or online.

Per Serving: Calories: 94; Protein: 7g; Cholesterol: 0mg; Sodium: 354mg; Total Carbohydrates: 10g; Fiber: 3g; Total Fat: 3g; Saturated Fat: 1g

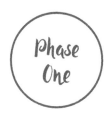

Phase One

PREP TIME: 5 MINUTES
COOK TIME: 15 MINUTES

1 (15-ounce) can
   low-sodium black beans,
   rinsed and drained

¼ teaspoon freshly ground
   black pepper, divided

¼ cup shredded
   Parmesan cheese

2 teaspoons extra-virgin
   olive oil, divided

4 cups sliced and stemmed
   kale leaves

¼ teaspoon salt, divided

4 eggs

4 tablespoons Fermented
   Salsa (page 217) or
   store-bought salsa

Fried Eggs over Greens and Beans

GRAIN-FREE | NUT-FREE | UNDER 30 MINUTES

Refried-style beans topped with eggs for breakfast? Yes! Though you may never have thought to serve beans at breakfast, they are a quick and easy way to get plenty of fiber and protein into your body first thing in the morning. Similar to making refried beans, but using no added fat, the black beans are roughly mashed and topped with a blanket of kale. Make sure the fried egg yolk is runny, as it forms a delicious, savory dressing when mixed with the beans and kale. SERVES 4

1. In a small pot, combine the beans and ½ cup of water. Bring to a boil over medium-high heat and simmer for 5 minutes. Mash the beans coarsely. Stir in ⅛ teaspoon of pepper and the Parmesan. Transfer to a dish and cover to keep warm.

2. In a large skillet, heat 1 teaspoon of olive oil over medium heat. Add the kale and ⅛ teaspoon of salt and stir to coat. Reduce the heat to medium-low and cook, stirring regularly, for 3 to 5 minutes, until the kale wilts. Remove from the heat and transfer to a plate.

3. Heat the remaining 1 teaspoon of olive oil in the pan over medium-high heat. Crack the eggs into the pan and fry for 3 to 5 minutes. For a firmer egg, cook for a bit longer; for a runnier egg, do not flip. Season with the remaining 1/8 teaspoon of salt and 1/8 teaspoon of pepper.

4. On each plate, arrange a scoop of beans, followed by a scoop of greens, and top with an egg. Add 1 tablespoon of salsa to each plate and serve.

Per Serving: Calories: 269; Protein: 19g; Cholesterol: 212mg; Sodium: 505mg; Total Carbohydrates: 28g; Fiber: 11g; Total Fat: 10g; Saturated Fat: 3g

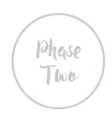
Phase Two

PREP TIME: 10 MINUTES
COOK TIME: 5 MINUTES

FOR THE PESTO

2 cups roughly torn
   kale leaves

2 tablespoons extra-virgin
   olive oil

¼ cup walnut pieces

2 garlic cloves

2 tablespoons grated
   Parmesan cheese

¼ teaspoon salt

Freshly ground
   black pepper

FOR THE EGGS

1 tablespoon white vinegar

4 eggs

Nonstick cooking spray

1 large tomato, diced

Poached Eggs on a Bed of Kale Pesto and Tomatoes

GRAIN-FREE | UNDER 30 MINUTES

The vibrant color and savory flavor of these eggs and greens will satisfy children and adults alike. Prepare the pesto up to three days in advance so you can make this dish quickly in the morning. **SERVES 2**

TO MAKE THE PESTO

In a blender, combine the kale, olive oil, walnuts, garlic, Parmesan, salt, and pepper. Process until smooth.

TO MAKE THE EGGS

1. In a small saucepan, bring about 3 inches of water to a simmer over medium-high heat. Add the vinegar.

2. Crack the eggs into the pan, one at a time, using a spoon each time to help hold the whites together slightly until they begin to firm. Cook for 3 to 5 minutes, depending on how runny you want the yolk. When cooked to your desired firmness, use a slotted spoon to remove the eggs from the pan.

3. Spray a small skillet with cooking spray and place over medium-high heat. Sauté the tomato briefly, until warmed through, then divide it between two serving plates. Top each with two poached eggs and a generous scoop of pesto. Serve.

MAKE AHEAD The pesto for this recipe can be made up to three days ahead. Store it in an airtight container until ready for use. If there is extra left over after making this recipe, use it as a seasoning to flavor vegetables, fish, or even salads.

Per Serving: Calories: 453; Protein: 22g; Cholesterol: 421mg; Sodium: 561mg; Total Carbohydrates: 14g; Fiber: 5g; Total Fat: 37g; Saturated Fat: 7g

Brown Rice and Egg Breakfast Bowl with Kimchi

DAIRY-FREE | NUT-FREE | UNDER 30 MINUTES

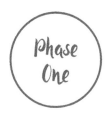

Phase One

Around the world, rice is commonly served at breakfast. Loaded with fiber and vitamins, brown rice is a filling grain that maintains its original bran layers, giving you all its nutrients. Brown rice has a shorter shelf life than its processed white counterparts, so you should purchase it in smaller quantities as needed to ensure its freshness. **SERVES 4**

1. Add ½ cup of rice to each of four bowls.

2. In a large skillet, heat the olive oil over medium-high heat. Crack the eggs into the skillet and fry them for 3 to 5 minutes. For a firmer egg, cook a bit longer and flip; for a runnier egg, do not flip. Season with the salt and pepper. Transfer 1 egg to each rice bowl.

3. Arrange ½ cup of kimchi, one-quarter of the avocado, and one-quarter of the scallions in each bowl.

4. In a small bowl, whisk the rice vinegar and sesame oil together and drizzle over each egg bowl. Serve.

PREP TIME: 10 MINUTES
COOK TIME: 5 MINUTES

2 cups cooked brown rice (see Tip)

1 teaspoon extra-virgin olive oil

4 eggs

Salt

Freshly ground black pepper

2 cups Kimchi with Sesame Seeds (page 214)

1 avocado, pitted, peeled, and cut into strips

4 scallions, green parts only, thinly sliced

¼ cup rice vinegar

1 teaspoon sesame oil

INGREDIENT TIP Several recipes in this book call for cooked brown rice. Here's how to cook it perfectly: For each cup of brown rice, use 2 cups of water and a pinch of salt. Combine in a saucepan and bring to a boil over medium-high heat. When it boils, reduce the heat to low, cover the pan, and simmer the rice for 45 minutes, until all the water has been absorbed. Fluff with a fork and enjoy.

Per Serving: Calories: 305; Protein: 11g; Cholesterol: 208mg; Sodium: 867mg; Total Carbohydrates: 30g; Fiber: 6g; Total Fat: 16g; Saturated Fat: 3g

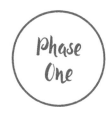

Phase One

PREP TIME: 10 MINUTES
COOK TIME: 25 MINUTES

Nonstick cooking spray

¼ cup gluten-free
  rolled oats

½ cup almond meal

¼ cup flaxseed meal

½ teaspoon
  ground cinnamon

1½ teaspoons
  baking powder

1 teaspoon salt

1 cup cooked quinoa

2 tablespoons canola oil

½ cup unsweetened
  applesauce

1 egg

1 teaspoon pure
  vanilla extract

½ cup golden raisins

Quinoa Almond Muffins

DAIRY-FREE

Quinoa muffins are a go-to breakfast item. Have one with a poached egg to stay powered up until lunchtime. Made with a blend of almond and oat flours, these gluten-free muffins pack in the protein and are sweetened with golden raisins and applesauce. **MAKES 12 MUFFINS**

1. Preheat the oven to 350°F.

2. Spray the cups of a muffin tin with cooking spray.

3. In a blender, process the oats until they are finely ground and resemble flour.

4. In a medium mixing bowl, combine the processed oats, almond meal, flaxseed meal, cinnamon, baking powder, and salt. Add the quinoa and mix to incorporate.

5. In a small bowl, mix the canola oil, applesauce, egg, and vanilla. Fold into the dry ingredients and stir until just mixed. Fold in the golden raisins.

6. Divide the batter between the 12 cups of the muffin tin, filling each about halfway. Bake for 25 minutes, until firm to the touch and lightly browned. Serve, or freeze in an airtight container for up to 1 month.

Per Serving: Calories: 158; Protein: 5g; Cholesterol: 17mg; Sodium: 249mg; Total Carbohydrates: 15g; Fiber: 3g; Total Fat: 10g; Saturated Fat: 1g

Apricot Nut Muffins

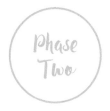

Apricots provide lovely nuggets of sweetness through-out these nutty muffins, while applesauce provides added flavor to the batter. Using a combination of oat and almond flours, these gluten-free muffins are filling on their own and even better when served with an egg. **MAKES 12 MUFFINS**

PREP TIME: 10 MINUTES
COOK TIME: 25 MINUTES

Nonstick cooking spray

2½ cups gluten-free rolled oats

½ cup almond flour

1½ teaspoons baking powder

1 teaspoon salt

1½ cups unsweetened plain yogurt or Kefir (page 211), or store-bought

½ cup unsweetened applesauce

2 eggs

2 tablespoons canola oil

½ cup diced dried apricots

¼ cup chopped walnuts

1. Preheat the oven to 350°F.

2. Spray the cups of a muffin tin with cooking spray.

3. In a blender, process the oats until they are finely ground and resemble flour.

4. In a mixing bowl, combine the processed oats, almond flour, baking powder, and salt.

5. In a small bowl, mix the yogurt, applesauce, eggs, and canola oil. Fold this mixture into the dry ingredients and stir until just mixed. Fold in the apricots and walnuts.

6. Divide the batter between the 12 cups of the muffin tin, filling each about halfway. Bake for 25 minutes, until firm to the touch and lightly browned. Serve, or freeze in an airtight container for up to 1 month.

INGREDIENT TIP Dried apricots are often dried unsweetened, unlike many other dried fruits, such as cranberries, which are so often sweetened. If desired, you can substitute any other type of unsweetened dried stone fruit, such as peaches, mangos, or nectarines, for the apricots.

Per Serving: Calories: 294; Protein: 12g; Cholesterol: 38mg; Sodium: 280mg; Total Carbohydrates: 30g; Fiber: 6g; Total Fat: 16g; Saturated Fat: 3g

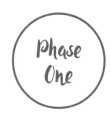

PREP TIME: 10 MINUTES
COOK TIME: 20 MINUTES

Nonstick cooking spray

½ cup smooth
   peanut butter

1 ripe banana, mashed

¼ cup honey

¼ cup unsweetened
   cocoa powder

2 tablespoons
   flaxseed meal

1 teaspoon pure
   vanilla extract

½ teaspoon baking soda

1 cup shredded zucchini

Chocolate, Peanut Butter, *and* Zucchini Muffins

DAIRY-FREE

Zucchini wonderfully adds vegetable bulk to muffins while its mild flavor is guided by whatever you mix with it. Here it meets up with chocolate, peanut butter, and an oat-almond flour mix that is sure to leave you satisfied and nourished. **MAKES 12 MUFFINS**

1. Preheat the oven to 375°F.

2. Spray the cups of a muffin tin with cooking spray.

3. In a large bowl, combine the peanut butter, banana, and honey. Mix well. Add the cocoa powder, flaxseed meal, and vanilla and stir to combine.

4. Sprinkle the baking soda over the mixture and stir to combine. Fold in the zucchini.

5. Divide the batter between the 12 cups of the muffin tin, filling each about halfway. Bake for 20 minutes, until firm to the touch and lightly browned. Serve, or freeze in an airtight container for up to 1 month.

Per Serving: Calories: 107; Protein: 4g; Cholesterol: 0mg; Sodium: 104mg; Total Carbohydrates: 12g; Fiber: 2g; Total Fat: 6g; Saturated Fat: 1g

Oat, Walnut, and Golden Raisin Granola

DAIRY-FREE

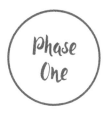

PREP TIME: 5 MINUTES
COOK TIME: 1 HOUR

For a quick breakfast, granola is the best. Store-bought varieties are loaded with sugar, but this simple home-made recipe tastes great without adding any. Mix it with yogurt and fresh fruit for a sweet and savory breakfast you can feel good about. Be sure to set the timer when you are cooking granola, as it can burn easily if not stirred regularly. **MAKES 2½ CUPS**

2 cups gluten-free rolled oats

½ cup walnut pieces

¼ cup sesame seeds

1 tablespoon ground cinnamon

1 teaspoon ground ginger

½ teaspoon salt

3 egg whites

¼ cup golden raisins

1. Preheat the oven to 225°F.

2. Line a baking sheet with parchment paper.

3. In a large bowl, mix the oats, walnuts, sesame seeds, cinnamon, ginger, and salt.

4. In a small bowl, beat the egg whites until well mixed, then fold them into the oats until well coated.

5. Transfer the oat mixture to the baking sheet and bake for 1 hour, stirring the granola every 20 minutes.

6. Remove from the oven and set aside to cool. Stir in the raisins. This granola can be stored in an airtight container for up to 2 weeks.

Per Serving (¼ cup): Calories: 200; Protein: 8g; Cholesterol: 0mg; Sodium: 132mg; Total Carbohydrates: 26g; Fiber: 5g; Total Fat: 8g; Saturated Fat: 1g

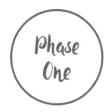

Phase One

PREP TIME: 5 MINUTES

2 cups gluten-free
  rolled oats

¼ cup almonds, broken
  into pieces

¼ cup cashews

¼ cup golden raisins

2 tablespoons flaxseed

½ cup unsweetened dried
  coconut flakes

Unsweetened plain
  dairy-free milk or
  unsweetened plain
  yogurt, for serving

Fresh raspberries,
  for serving

Oat *and* Nut Muesli *with* Raspberries

UNDER 30 MINUTES

Muesli is similar to granola, except that it's not cooked. Instead, this quick cereal-like mixture is simply combined and stored until ready to eat. Because it's dry, it's best served mixed into a bowl of yogurt or with dairy-free milk, such as almond, hemp, or soy milk. **MAKES 2½ CUPS**

1. In a mixing bowl, combine the oats, almonds, cashews, raisins, flaxseed, and coconut. Stir well to combine and transfer to an airtight container.

2. To serve, place ½ cup of muesli in a bowl and pour ½ cup of nondairy milk over it. Top with raspberries. Store the muesli in an airtight container for up to 2 weeks.

Per Serving: Calories: 216; Protein: 8g; Cholesterol: 0mg; Sodium: 4mg; Total Carbohydrates: 28g; Fiber: 5g; Total Fat: 9g; Saturated Fat: 3g

Probiotic Cinnamon Steel Cut Oats

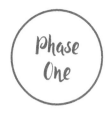

PREP TIME: 5 MINUTES
COOK TIME: 25 MINUTES

Steel cut oats are a bit firmer than rolled oats and have a rather pleasing texture. Cut from whole oat groats, they have a shorter cooking time than when whole and are less processed than rolled oats. Here they are mixed with cinnamon, flaxseed, kefir, and vanilla for a tasty probiotic powerhouse. **SERVES 4**

1 cup gluten-free steel cut oats

¼ teaspoon salt

2 tablespoons flaxseed meal

1 cup Kefir (page 211), or store-bought

1½ teaspoons ground cinnamon

1 teaspoon pure vanilla extract

4 tablespoons walnut pieces

4 tablespoons golden raisins

1. In a medium pot, bring the oats, salt, flaxseed meal, and 3 cups of water to a boil over high heat. Boil for 1 minute, reduce the heat to low, and simmer for 25 minutes.

2. Remove the oatmeal from the heat and stir in the kefir, cinnamon, and vanilla. Divide between four bowls, top each with 1 tablespoon each of walnuts and raisins, and serve.

Per Serving: Calories: 296; Protein: 12g; Cholesterol: 3mg; Sodium: 170mg; Total Carbohydrates: 43g; Fiber: 7g; Total Fat: 10g; Saturated Fat: 2g

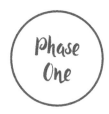

Phase One

PREP TIME: 5 MINUTES
COOK TIME: 20 MINUTES

⅓ cup gluten-free
rolled oats

⅓ cup unsweetened plain
almond milk

⅓ cup unsweetened
plain yogurt

2 teaspoons chia seeds

½ cup fresh fruit
(strawberries, bananas,
blueberries, raspberries,
grapes, peaches, plums)

Overnight Oatmeal
with **Fruit** and **Nuts**

UNDER 30 MINUTES

Make a couple of these every week to have on hand for a morning when you would rather not think about breakfast, and you will be a happier person. So easy to make, and so delicious, these simple breakfast cups are perfect for busy work mornings. If you prefer, toss it in the microwave with a little extra almond milk to serve hot, or eat it right out of the fridge. SERVES 1

In a small jar, mix the oats, almond milk, yogurt, and chia seeds together. Cover and refrigerate overnight. Stir and top with your choice of fresh fruit. Premade jars of oatmeal may be stored in the refrigerator for 3 to 4 days.

Per Serving: Calories: 351; Protein: 15g; Cholesterol: 13mg; Sodium: 120mg;
Total Carbohydrates: 51g; Fiber: 11g; Total Fat: 11g; Saturated Fat: 3g

Yogurt Parfait

UNDER 30 MINUTES

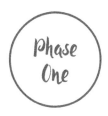

PREP TIME: 5 MINUTES

Yogurt parfaits take just minutes to throw together and are just as easy to enjoy. Mix and match your favorite fruits in this recipe, and you have a customizable breakfast that doesn't get old. Prepare a couple of these at once to cut down on prep time and have extras on hand for when you don't feel like making breakfast. **SERVES 2**

2 cups unsweetened plain yogurt

2 teaspoons pure vanilla extract

½ cup Oat, Walnut, and Golden Raisin Granola (page 85), divided

½ cup sliced fresh strawberries

½ cup fresh blueberries

1. In a small bowl, mix the yogurt and vanilla.

2. Scoop ½ cup of the yogurt mixture into each of two small cups. Top each with 2 tablespoons of granola, strawberries, and blueberries.

3. Add another ½ cup of the yogurt mixture to each cup and top with the remaining granola and fruit.

MAKE AHEAD These can be made up to three days in advance. Cover with an airtight lid and store in the refrigerator.

Per Serving: Calories: 405; Protein: 17g; Cholesterol: 35mg; Sodium: 283mg; Total Carbohydrates: 49g; Fiber: 6g; Total Fat: 16g; Saturated Fat: 6g

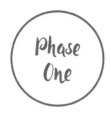

PREP TIME: 5 MINUTES

¼ cup chia seeds

1 cup unsweetened plain yogurt

1 small honeydew or cantaloupe melon, halved and seeded

1 kiwi fruit, peeled and sliced

½ cup fresh blueberries

½ cup fresh raspberries

¼ cup sliced almonds

Chia Yogurt Melon Bowl

GRAIN-FREE | UNDER 30 MINUTES

No need to break out the dishes when you eat a melon breakfast bowl—the melon actually works as the bowl. You can prep these the night before if desired; just make sure that you drain any excess juice from the melon so that the contents do not get soggy. **SERVES 2**

In a small bowl, mix the chia seeds and yogurt. Divide the mixture between the two melon halves. Top with kiwi slices, blueberries, raspberries, and almonds. Serve.

Per Serving: Calories: 533; Protein: 15g; Cholesterol: 18mg; Sodium: 173mg; Total Carbohydrates: 82g; Fiber: 21g; Total Fat: 20g; Saturated Fat: 4g

Vanilla Chia Seed Pudding *with* Strawberries *and* Almonds

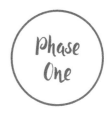

Phase One

DAIRY-FREE | GRAIN-FREE | VEGAN | UNDER 30 MINUTES

PREP TIME: 5 MINUTES

Topped with fruit and nuts, this no-cook, protein-rich pudding is a perfect dish to get you going in the morning. Gelatinous chia seeds thicken the almond milk overnight to create a simple pudding. Mix the chia and milk at least an hour before you are ready to serve and top with fresh strawberries and almonds. **SERVES 2**

½ cup chia seeds

2 cups unsweetened plain almond milk

2 teaspoons pure vanilla extract

¼ cup sliced almonds

1 cup sliced fresh strawberries

1. In each of two small containers or cups, mix ¼ cup of chia seeds and 1 cup of almond milk. Add 1 teaspoon of vanilla to each cup. Stir well, cover, and refrigerate overnight.

2. In the morning, stir to incorporate. Top with the almonds and strawberries, and serve.

MAKE AHEAD Make these up to three days in advance. Before serving, stir well to mix the chia seeds throughout the pudding and top with fruit, nuts, or seeds, as desired.

Per Serving: Calories: 438; Protein: 14g; Cholesterol: 0mg; Sodium: 193mg; Total Carbohydrates: 38g; Fiber: 27g; Total Fat: 28g; Saturated Fat: 3g

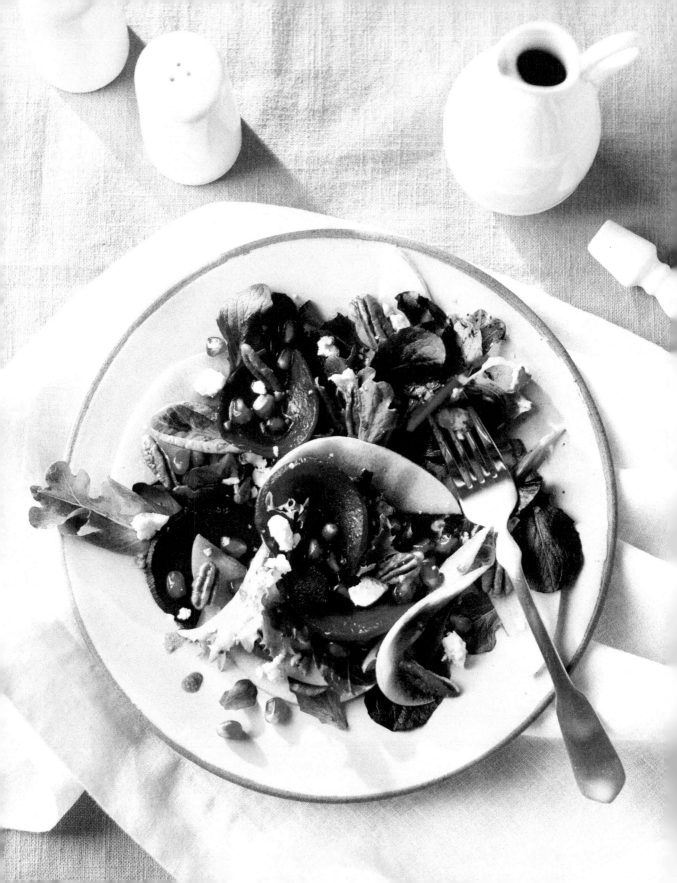

Soups, Stews, and Salads

Soups and salads can form a meal on their own, or they can be served as a side dish to a larger meal. Either way, you will be winning when it comes to adding more vegetables to your diet. Soups and salads are often perfect for making ahead of time, and are flexible in that they can be mixed and matched with a wide variety of meals. The flexibility to mix and match makes them seem luxurious when compared with the short amount of time you will spend preparing them.

Beet Yogurt Soup

GRAIN-FREE | NUT-FREE

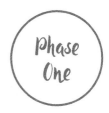

Phase One

Beets are packed with vitamins and minerals, which give them their striking red color. This soup is simple and clean, livened with a scoop of yogurt at the end to pack in some extra probiotic goodness. Be sure that you remove the soup from the heat before adding the yogurt so that the heat does not destroy the valuable living bacteria—and it's best served right after you make it, rather than stored and reheated, for the same reason. SERVES 4 TO 6

PREP TIME: 5 MINUTES
COOK TIME: 35 MINUTES

4 medium beets

1 potato, peeled

2 celery stalks, roughly chopped

1 yellow onion, peeled

1 cup packed spinach leaves

2 cups low-sodium vegetable broth

½ teaspoon salt

¼ teaspoon freshly ground black pepper

½ cup unsweetened plain yogurt

1. Fill a medium saucepan with about 2 inches of water and place the pan over medium-high heat.

2. In a steamer basket, place the beets, potato, celery, and onion. Put the basket in the saucepan (making sure the water does not touch the vegetables) and bring the water to a boil. Cover the pan and steam the vegetables for 30 minutes, until the beets are tender when pierced with a fork. Add the spinach to the basket and steam until just wilted.

3. Remove all the vegetables from the basket and transfer them to a blender. Process until smooth and place back in the empty saucepan.

4. Add the broth, salt, and pepper and bring to a simmer over medium heat for 5 minutes. Remove from the heat and add the yogurt, whisking to combine. Serve.

DID YOU KNOW? Beets get their color from the pigment betalain, the same component that makes varieties of Swiss chard red. Because of the vegetable's inherent sweetness, the sugar beet, a relative of the common red beet, is specifically grown for and processed into sugar, accounting for up to one-third of worldwide sugar production.

Per Serving: Calories: 144; Protein: 4g; Cholesterol: 3mg; Sodium: 483mg; Total Carbohydrates: 23g; Fiber: 6g; Total Fat: 4g; Saturated Fat: 1g

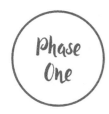

Phase One

PREP TIME: 5 MINUTES
COOK TIME: 10 MINUTES

1 tablespoon dried wakame seaweed flakes (see Tip)

4 cups low-sodium vegetable stock

½ cup cubed firm tofu

2 tablespoons miso paste

2 tablespoons chopped scallions, white and green parts

Miso Soup with Tofu and Seaweed

DAIRY-FREE | NUT-FREE | VEGAN | UNDER 30 MINUTES

A cornerstone of the Japanese diet, miso soup fits nicely into the microbiome diet as well. Made using the fermented soy product miso, this salty soup is nourishing and delicious. This soup can be served as any meal of the day—including breakfast, as it is in Japan—or as a light accompaniment. Serve it hot right after you make it, as it cannot be stored. While traditional miso uses a dashi fish stock, this version substitutes vegetable stock to make it more accessible. You will need to source some miso paste, which can be found in many well-stocked grocery stores and most Asian markets. Look for shiro, or white, miso, which has a lighter flavor than other varieties and is perfect for miso soup. SERVES 4

1. In a small bowl, cover the wakame with cool water and set it aside.

2. In a small saucepan, heat the vegetable stock over medium-high heat until simmering. Add the tofu and heat through.

3. Drain the wakame, squeezing out the excess water. Add it to the stock and stir. Turn off the heat.

4. Place the miso paste in a large ladle, and add a bit of the stock to the ladle. Use a chopstick or fork to mix the miso and stock together. While mixing, pour the liquid back into the saucepan, scoop up a bit more stock, and repeat until all the miso is mixed in, without any lumps.

5. Divide the soup into four bowls and top with the scallions. Serve.

INGREDIENT TIP Wakame is an olive-green sea vegetable hailing predominately from Northern Japan. It is rich in calcium, iron, protein, and niacin, as well as vitamins A and C. Look for it at any Asian market, where it is readily available.

TIP Removing the soup from the heat before adding the miso prevents the heat from destroying the valuable living bacteria.

Per Serving: Calories: 39; Protein: 3g; Cholesterol: 0mg; Sodium: 419mg; Total Carbohydrates: 4g; Fiber: 1g; Total Fat: 1g; Saturated Fat: 0g

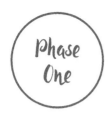

Phase One

PREP TIME: 5 MINUTES
COOK TIME: 20 MINUTES

¼ cup extra-virgin olive oil

1 large yellow onion, cut into wedges

2 (28-ounce) cans whole low-sodium tomatoes

1 teaspoon salt

¼ teaspoon freshly ground black pepper

1 cup unsweetened plain almond milk

Creamy Tomato Soup

DAIRY-FREE | GRAIN-FREE | VEGAN | UNDER 30 MINUTES

Tomato soup is a classic comfort food. Skip the stuff from a can that is laden with preservatives and sugar, and instead make this warming, simple soup in just minutes. By using canned tomatoes, you can cut out much of the prep work and have soup on the table in a flash. **SERVES 4 TO 6**

1. In a large saucepan, heat the olive oil over medium-high heat. Add the onion and cook for 2 to 3 minutes, until fragrant.

2. Add the tomatoes and their juices along with 2 cups of water to the saucepan. Bring to a simmer, reduce the heat to medium-low, and simmer for 20 minutes, stirring occasionally.

3. Using an immersion blender or blender, purée the soup to the desired consistency. If using a blender, work in batches to prevent splattering, as the soup is hot.

4. Add the salt, pepper, and almond milk. Stir to heat through, and serve.

INGREDIENT TIP Canned tomatoes have the most flavor when they are canned whole. If available, look for a variety that is fire-roasted, which locks in even more flavor.

MAKE AHEAD This soup can be made up to three days in advance and stored in the refrigerator.

Per Serving: Calories: 212; Protein: 4g; Cholesterol: 0mg; Sodium: 904mg; Total Carbohydrates: 20g; Fiber: 5g; Total Fat: 15g; Saturated Fat: 2g

Simple Lentil Soup

DAIRY-FREE | GRAIN-FREE | NUT-FREE | VEGAN

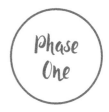

Phase One

PREP TIME: 10 MINUTES
COOK TIME: 40 MINUTES

A cup of good lentil soup is warming, filling, and loaded with fiber and vegetables. While many versions of lentil soup use smoked meat to add flavor, this one is vegetable driven and complex. Make a double batch if you like it, as it freezes well and is a great consolation on a cold and blustery day. **SERVES 4**

1. In a large pot, heat the olive oil over medium-high heat. Add the onion, celery, and carrots and cook, stirring frequently, for about 5 minutes, until the vegetables are lightly browned. Add the garlic and cook for 1 minute, stirring continuously.

2. Add the lentils, broth, tomatoes, cumin, coriander, salt, and pepper and bring to a boil. Reduce the heat and simmer for 20 to 25 minutes, until the lentils are soft. Add the chard and continue simmering for 10 minutes more, until the lentils are tender and the soup has thickened.

3. Add the lemon juice to the soup and stir to combine. Serve.

MAKE AHEAD Freeze this soup for up to 1 month in an airtight container. To serve, thaw in the refrigerator overnight and reheat in a saucepan on the stove or in a microwave-safe dish in the microwave.

Per Serving: Calories: 302; Protein: 14g; Cholesterol: 0mg; Sodium: 581mg; Total Carbohydrates: 43g; Fiber: 19g; Total Fat: 8g; Saturated Fat: 1g

2 tablespoons extra-virgin olive oil

1 yellow onion, diced

2 celery stalks, diced

2 carrots, diced

4 garlic cloves, minced

1 cup brown or French green lentils, picked over and rinsed

4 cups low-sodium vegetable broth

1 (15-ounce) can diced tomatoes, drained

½ teaspoon ground cumin

½ teaspoon ground coriander

½ teaspoon salt

¼ teaspoon freshly ground black pepper

1 cup chopped Swiss chard

Juice of 1 lemon

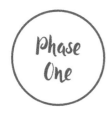

Phase One

PREP TIME: 10 MINUTES
COOK TIME: 25 MINUTES

2 tablespoons extra-virgin
   olive oil

1 yellow onion, diced

4 parsnips, diced

2 garlic cloves, minced

2 tablespoons
   curry powder

4 cups low-sodium
   vegetable broth

½ cup red lentils, picked
   over and rinsed

½ teaspoon salt

Juice of ½ lemon

¼ cup roughly chopped
   cilantro, for serving

Unsweetened plain yogurt,
   for serving

Curried Lentil and Parsnip Soup

GRAIN-FREE | NUT-FREE

This curried lentil soup is a warming twist on the ordinary. Parsnips add richness to the soup, which is puréed and served with a generous dollop of yogurt on top. Red lentils give this lightly spiced soup a bright hue. **SERVES 4**

1. In a large saucepan, heat the olive oil over medium-high heat. Add the onion and parsnips, and cook, stirring frequently, for about 5 minutes, until the vegetables are lightly browned. Add the garlic and cook for 1 minute, stirring constantly.

2. Add the curry powder and stir for an additional minute, until fragrant. Add the broth and bring to a boil. Reduce the heat, add the lentils and salt, and simmer for 20 minutes, until the lentils are tender.

3. Purée the soup in batches using a blender, or use an immersion blender to purée it directly in the pot. Stir in the lemon juice. Serve, topped with the cilantro and a dollop of yogurt.

MAKE AHEAD Freeze this soup for up to 1 month in an airtight container. To serve, thaw in the refrigerator overnight and reheat in a saucepan on the stove or in a microwave-safe dish in the microwave.

Per Serving: Calories: 226; Protein: 7g; Cholesterol: 0mg; Sodium: 441mg; Total Carbohydrates: 33g; Fiber: 12g; Total Fat: 8g; Saturated Fat: 1g

Simple Black Bean Soup

GRAIN-FREE | NUT-FREE | UNDER 30 MINUTES

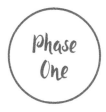

Phase One

Thick and spicy, this black bean soup is a creamy masterpiece when topped with a heaping spoonful of yogurt. Prepare a Simple Green Side Salad (page 107) while the soup is cooking, and you have a balanced and tasty meal in less than 30 minutes from start to finish. Perfect. **SERVES 4**

PREP TIME: 5 MINUTES
COOK TIME: 15 MINUTES

1. In a large saucepan, heat the olive oil over medium-high heat. Sauté the onion and green pepper for about 5 minutes, until they begin to soften. Add the garlic and stir for 1 minute.

2. Add the beans, broth, vinegar, cumin, salt, and pepper. Bring to a boil, reduce the heat, and simmer for 10 minutes. Serve with a dollop of yogurt and garnished with the cilantro.

MAKE AHEAD Freeze this soup for up to 1 month in an airtight container. To serve, thaw in the refrigerator overnight and reheat in a saucepan on the stove or in a microwave-safe dish in the microwave.

Per Serving: Calories: 288; Protein: 4g; Cholesterol: 0mg; Sodium: 765mg; Total Carbohydrates: 48g; Fiber: 19g; Total Fat: 4g; Saturated Fat: 1g

1 tablespoon extra-virgin olive oil

1 large yellow onion, diced

1 small green bell pepper, stemmed, seeded, and diced

2 garlic cloves, minced

2 (15-ounce) cans low-sodium black beans, drained and rinsed

4 cups low-sodium vegetable broth

1 tablespoon white wine vinegar

1 teaspoon ground cumin

1 teaspoon salt

¼ teaspoon freshly ground black pepper

Unsweetened plain yogurt, for serving

Cilantro, for garnish

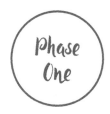

Phase One

PREP TIME: 5 MINUTES
COOK TIME: 15 MINUTES

1 tablespoon extra-virgin
   olive oil

1 small yellow onion, diced

2 (15-ounce) cans
   low-sodium black beans,
   drained and rinsed

1 (15-ounce) can
   fire-roasted tomatoes

1 chipotle chile in adobo
   sauce, finely minced

½ teaspoon salt

Freshly ground
   black pepper

Black Bean Chili

DAIRY-FREE | GRAIN-FREE | NUT-FREE | VEGAN | UNDER 30 MINUTES

Chili lovers will appreciate this simple, no-nonsense chili that tastes great. This quick version uses canned black beans to eliminate lengthy soaking and cooking time, and requires just a few ingredients to make a wonderful chili in a matter of minutes. SERVES 4

1. In a large saucepan, heat the olive oil over medium-high heat. Add the onion and sauté until it begins to soften, about 5 minutes.

2. Add the beans, tomatoes, and chipotle chile to the saucepan and stir to incorporate. Bring to a boil, reduce the heat, and simmer for 10 minutes. Season with salt and pepper to taste. Serve.

INGREDIENT TIP Look for chipotle chiles in adobo sauce in the Mexican section of your supermarket. One can will last you quite a while, as it contains multiple peppers. Once open, the best way to store them is to freeze them. Purée the whole can and freeze in ice cube trays, then transfer to a zip-top freezer storage bag once frozen solid. One ice cube–size piece equals about one pepper.

MAKE AHEAD This soup can be made up to three days in advance and stored in the refrigerator.

Per Serving: Calories: 324; Protein: 15g; Cholesterol: 0mg; Sodium: 707mg; Total Carbohydrates: 43g; Fiber: 18g; Total Fat: 11g; Saturated Fat: 2g

Chickpea, Tomato, and Kale Soup

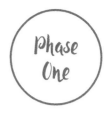

Phase One

DAIRY-FREE | GRAIN-FREE | NUT-FREE | VEGAN

Chickpeas are firmer than most beans, allowing them to hold their shape after cooking. Here they are center stage, providing protein and a nutty flavor that complements this simple tomato-infused soup. With the addition of plenty of leafy green kale, this is a well-balanced meal that will keep you full all afternoon long. **SERVES 4 TO 6**

PREP TIME: 10 MINUTES
COOK TIME: 25 MINUTES

1 tablespoon extra-virgin olive oil

1 medium yellow onion, diced

3 garlic cloves, minced

2 (15-ounce) cans low-sodium chickpeas

1 (15-ounce) can fire-roasted tomatoes

2 cups low-sodium vegetable broth

1 tablespoon smoked paprika

2 teaspoons ground turmeric

1 teaspoon dried oregano

1 teaspoon salt

½ teaspoon freshly ground black pepper

1 bunch kale, stemmed and thinly sliced

1. In a large saucepan, heat the olive oil over medium-high heat. Add the onion and cook, stirring regularly, for about 5 minutes, until it begins to soften. Add the garlic and cook for 1 minute more.

2. Add the chickpeas, tomatoes, broth, 2 cups of water, the paprika, turmeric, oregano, salt, and pepper. Stir well, bring to a boil, reduce the heat, and simmer for 20 minutes.

3. Stir in the kale and cook briefly, until just wilted. Remove from the heat and serve.

MAKE AHEAD Freeze this soup for up to 1 month in an airtight container. To serve, thaw in the refrigerator overnight and reheat in a saucepan on the stove or in a microwave-safe dish in the microwave.

Per Serving: Calories: 252; Protein: 11g; Cholesterol: 0mg; Sodium: 713mg; Total Carbohydrates: 39g; Fiber: 11g; Total Fat: 7g; Saturated Fat: 1g

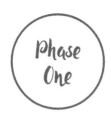

Phase One

PREP TIME: 10 MINUTES
COOK TIME: 35 MINUTES

1 tablespoon extra-virgin olive oil

2 yellow onions, diced

1 cup low-sodium vegetable broth

2 large russet potatoes, peeled and cut into 1-inch chunks

1 celery stalk, diced

1 teaspoon salt

2 cups frozen corn, thawed

1 cup unsweetened plain almond milk

¼ teaspoon freshly ground black pepper

1 pound cod fillets, cut into 1-inch pieces

Corn and Whitefish Chowder

DAIRY-FREE | GRAIN-FREE

Creamy soups are great comfort food, and sometimes you just need to indulge. This thick and rich chowder is perfect for the occasion but is actually guilt-free as it calls for almond milk instead of cream. Believe me, you won't miss the cream. Take the corn out of the freezer when you start making the soup, and it should be defrosted in time. **SERVES 4 TO 6**

1. In a large saucepan, heat the olive oil over medium-high heat. Add the onions and cook, stirring frequently, for about 5 minutes, until they have softened.

2. Add 2 cups of water, the broth, potatoes, celery, and salt. Bring to a boil, reduce the heat, and simmer for 20 minutes. Mash the mixture with a masher or use an immersion blender to purée.

3. Add the corn, almond milk, and pepper. Simmer for 5 minutes more.

4. Add the cod, bring the soup back to a simmer, and cook for 3 minutes, until the cod is just cooked and flakes easily when tested with a fork. Serve.

MAKE AHEAD This soup can be made up to three days in advance, and actually tastes better after a day in the refrigerator to allow the flavors to combine. Make it on the weekend and then have it later in the week to see if you can notice the difference in the flavor.

Per Serving: Calories: 354; Protein: 25g; Cholesterol: 53mg; Sodium: 745mg; Total Carbohydrates: 54g; Fiber: 5g; Total Fat: 6g; Saturated Fat: 1g

Chicken *and* Brown Rice Soup

DAIRY-FREE | NUT-FREE

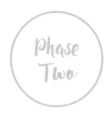

Phase Two

Chicken and rice soup is a classic comfort food that is so good, and so good for you. Loaded with brown rice and plenty of vegetables, this fiber- and vitamin-packed soup will keep you feeling full, well-nourished, and content. **SERVES 2 TO 4**

PREP TIME: 10 MINUTES
COOK TIME: 25 MINUTES

1 tablespoon extra-virgin olive oil

1 yellow onion, diced

2 celery stalks, diced

2 carrots, diced

4 garlic cloves, minced

1 (1-inch) piece ginger, peeled and minced

8 ounces boneless skinless chicken breasts, cut into ½-inch cubes

4 cups low-sodium chicken broth

1 cup cooked brown rice (see page 81)

½ teaspoon salt

¼ teaspoon freshly ground black pepper

1. In a large saucepan, heat the olive oil over medium-high heat. Add the onion, celery, and carrots and cook, stirring frequently, for about 5 minutes, until they have lightly browned. Add the garlic and ginger, and cook for 1 minute, stirring constantly.

2. Add the chicken to the pot and stir for 2 to 3 minutes, until the chicken is lightly browned. Add the chicken broth and bring to a boil. Reduce the heat and simmer for 10 minutes. Add the rice, salt, and pepper. Cook for 5 minutes more, until heated through. Serve.

MAKE AHEAD Freeze this soup for up to 1 month in an airtight container. To serve, thaw in the refrigerator overnight and reheat in a saucepan on the stove or in a microwave-safe dish in the microwave.

Per Serving: Calories: 205; Protein: 18g; Cholesterol: 30mg; Sodium: 517mg; Total Carbohydrates: 22g; Fiber: 3g; Total Fat: 6g; Saturated Fat: 1g

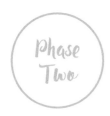

Phase Two

PREP TIME: 10 MINUTES
COOK TIME: 35 MINUTES

2 tablespoons canola
  oil, divided

1 pound boneless
  beef sirloin, cut into
  1-inch cubes

1 yellow onion, diced

2 garlic cloves, minced

2 carrots, diced

1 turnip, diced

1 parsnip, diced

4 cups low-sodium
  beef broth

½ teaspoon salt

½ teaspoon freshly ground
  black pepper

Beef and Root Vegetable Stew

DAIRY-FREE | GRAIN-FREE | NUT-FREE

You may think beef stew needs all afternoon to cook, but if you use tender cuts, you don't have to cook it for as long as traditional stew cuts of beef. In this quick stew, tender beef meets a mixture of root vegetables and is simply seasoned with just salt and pepper. The flavor is in the rich beef and trio of carrots, turnip, and parsnip that make up the bulk of this warming favorite. SERVES 4

1. In a large saucepan, heat 1 tablespoon of canola oil over medium-high heat. Add the beef and cook, stirring regularly, for 5 to 7 minutes, until the beef is well browned on all sides. Remove from the saucepan and set it aside.

2. Heat the remaining 1 tablespoon of oil over medium-high heat. Add the onion and cook, stirring frequently, for about 5 minutes, until it has lightly browned. Add the garlic and cook for 1 minute, stirring continuously.

3. Return the beef to the pan, along with the carrots, turnip, parsnip, and beef broth. Season with the salt and pepper. Bring to a boil, reduce the heat, and simmer for 20 minutes, until the vegetables are tender and the stew has thickened slightly. Serve.

MAKE AHEAD Freeze this stew for up to 1 month in an airtight container. To serve, thaw in the refrigerator overnight and reheat in a saucepan on the stove or in a microwave-safe dish in the microwave.

Per Serving: Calories: 370; Protein: 27g; Cholesterol: 85mg; Sodium: 779mg; Total Carbohydrates: 16g; Fiber: 4g; Total Fat: 22g; Saturated Fat: 6g

Simple Green Side Salad

DAIRY-FREE | GRAIN-FREE | NUT-FREE | VEGAN | UNDER 30 MINUTES

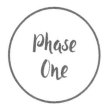

Salads can be as complex or as simple as you dream them up to be. While a salad loaded with vegetables, fruits, and nuts has its place, so does the simple bare-bones go-to weeknight salad. This one is so quick to put together that there's really no reason not to get that extra portion of veggies into your day. **SERVES 2 TO 4**

In a large bowl, toss together the lettuce, scallions, and carrot. Drizzle with your dressing of choice and toss again. Serve.

MAKE AHEAD Prep the vegetables for this salad up to 3 days in advance. To save time, wash and prep several heads of lettuce at once and store in an airtight container in the refrigerator to use throughout the week. When ready to serve, toss the salad with dressing.

INGREDIENT TIP All lettuce is not created equal. Romaine is a great go-to lettuce because its firmness allows you to prep it in advance without it wilting. Other good choices are green leaf lettuces such as Bibb and Buttercrunch. While the crunch of iceberg lettuce is part of its allure, try to avoid using it in salads, as many of its bitter properties, which are where the nutrients lie, have been bred out, leaving a nutritionally depleted lettuce.

Per Serving (with Skinny Caesar): Calories: 44; Protein: 2g; Cholesterol: 5mg; Sodium: 120mg; Total Carbohydrates: 6g; Fiber: 2g; Total Fat: 1g; Saturated Fat: 1g

PREP TIME: 5 MINUTES

1 medium head romaine lettuce (see Tip)

2 scallions, white and green parts, thinly sliced

1 carrot, shredded

Red Wine Vinaigrette (page 201), Blue Cheese Dressing (page 204), Skinny Caesar Dressing (page 205), Sesame-Ginger Dressing (page 108), or Bright Lemon-Garlic Vinaigrette (page 202)

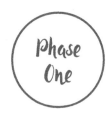

Phase One

PREP TIME: 10 MINUTES, PLUS 1 HOUR TO REST

FOR THE DRESSING

1 (1-inch) piece fresh ginger, minced

1 teaspoon sesame oil

2 tablespoons extra-virgin olive oil

2 tablespoons rice vinegar

¼ teaspoon salt

Freshly ground black pepper

FOR THE SALAD

1 bunch kale, stemmed and thinly sliced

2 carrots, shredded

4 scallions, green parts only, thinly sliced

Asian Kale Salad *with* Sesame-Ginger Dressing

DAIRY-FREE | GRAIN-FREE | NUT-FREE | VEGAN

Toss this salad together first before you make your entrée, and let it rest in the refrigerator for about an hour to allow the flavors to blend. It will taste even better the next day, if you can wait. Make a double batch to have plenty for quick meals during the upcoming week, and you will be glad you did. SERVES 4

TO MAKE THE DRESSING

In a small bowl, whisk the ginger, sesame oil, olive oil, rice vinegar, and salt. Season with pepper.

TO MAKE THE SALAD

1. In a large bowl, combine the kale, carrots, and scallions. Toss well.

2. Pour the dressing over the salad and use your clean hands to massage the dressing into the salad, making sure that it is evenly distributed. Cover and refrigerate for 1 hour before serving. Store refrigerated in an airtight container for 3 to 5 days.

INGREDIENT TIP Be sure to slice the kale thinly, which allows it to take on more of the dressing. Curly kale varieties work great when you are going to cook the kale, but for a fresh kale salad, Lacinato kale, also known as Tuscan and dinosaur kale, works best.

Per Serving: Calories: 126; Protein: 2g; Cholesterol: 0mg; Sodium: 456mg; Total Carbohydrates: 12g; Fiber: 3g; Total Fat: 8g; Saturated Fat: 1g

Fragrant Fennel *and* Kohlrabi Salad

DAIRY-FREE | GRAIN-FREE | VEGAN | UNDER 30 MINUTES

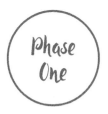

Fennel, the wonderfully fragrant winter vegetable, shows up in stores in the fall and remains throughout the winter until spring. It's combined with another fall and winter favorite, kohlrabi, in this quick-to-prepare salad. Lightly seasoned with just olive oil and lemon juice, it is simple, refreshing, and delivers a sprightly crunch. And it holds up well to refrigeration, making it a good make-ahead salad choice. **SERVES 4**

In a large bowl, toss together the fennel and kohlrabi. Sprinkle with the salt and pepper and toss again. Add the olive oil and lemon juice, and mix to combine. Fold in the walnuts and serve.

MAKE AHEAD Toss the salad, with everything but the walnuts, and store refrigerated in an airtight container for up to 3 days before serving. To serve, top with the walnuts.

Per Serving: Calories: 137; Protein: 2g; Cholesterol: 0mg; Sodium: 183mg; Total Carbohydrates: 8g; Fiber: 4g; Total Fat: 12g; Saturated Fat: 1g

PREP TIME: 10 MINUTES

1 large fennel bulb, trimmed and thinly sliced

1 small kohlrabi bulb, peeled, trimmed, and cut into matchsticks

¼ teaspoon salt

¼ teaspoon freshly ground black pepper

2 tablespoons extra-virgin olive oil

Juice of 1 lemon

¼ cup chopped walnuts

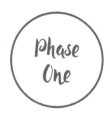

PREP TIME: 15 MINUTES, PLUS 2 HOURS TO CHILL

2 large tomatoes, seeded and diced

1 large cucumber, peeled and diced

1 green bell pepper, seeded and diced

1 shallot, diced

½ cup sliced kalamata olives

2 tablespoons extra-virgin olive oil

2 tablespoons red wine vinegar

½ teaspoon salt

¼ teaspoon freshly ground black pepper

1 garlic clove, minced

2 scallions, white and green parts, thinly sliced

Gazpacho Salad

DAIRY-FREE | GRAIN-FREE | NUT-FREE | VEGAN

Cold tomato gazpacho soup tastes just as good in salad form. In this cubed remake, a blend of tomatoes, cucumber, green pepper, shallot, and olives marinate in a vinegar-and-oil blend to create a refreshing side dish. There is no need to go crazy getting all the tomato seeds out. Try cutting the tomato in quarters and scraping out the seed cavities before dicing to eliminate tedious knife work. SERVES 4 TO 6

1. In a large bowl, toss the tomatoes, cucumber, bell pepper, shallot, and olives.

2. In a small bowl, whisk the olive oil, vinegar, salt, pepper, and garlic. Pour the dressing over the vegetable mixture and toss to combine. Cover and refrigerate for 2 hours. Toss again before serving, topped with the scallions.

Per Serving: Calories: 147; Protein: 2g; Cholesterol: 0mg; Sodium: 278mg; Total Carbohydrates: 10g; Fiber: 2g; Total Fat: 12g; Saturated Fat: 1g

Sweet *and* Savory Orange Walnut Salad

GRAIN-FREE | UNDER 30 MINUTES

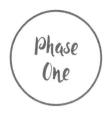

Phase One

Mandarin oranges are used to add a citrus punch to this salad that mixes sweet and savory flavors. While fresh mandarins are best, you could also substitute a can of them; just be sure to look for ones that are canned with no added sugar. SERVES 4

PREP TIME: 10 MINUTES

8 cups salad greens

½ cup walnut pieces

3 mandarin oranges, peeled and separated into segments

½ cup crumbled blue cheese (see Tip)

¼ cup Red Wine Vinaigrette (page 201)

1. In a large bowl, toss the salad greens, walnuts, oranges, and blue cheese.

2. Drizzle the dressing over the salad and toss to combine. Serve.

INGREDIENT TIP Blue cheese comes in many varieties, making this salad customizable to your own tastes. If you are not a lover of blue cheese, try milder varieties such as Gorgonzola or Danish blue in this salad. If you like the distinctive bite and aroma of blue cheese, try a stronger-tasting variety such as Roquefort.

Per Serving: Calories: 280; Protein: 7g; Cholesterol: 13mg; Sodium: 339mg; Total Carbohydrates: 13g; Fiber: 3g; Total Fat: 24g; Saturated Fat: 5g

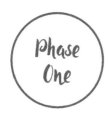

Phase One

PREP TIME: 10 MINUTES
COOK TIME: 25 MINUTES

2 medium beets

3 cups mixed salad greens

1 pear (Seckel, Comice, Bartlett), cored and thinly sliced lengthwise

Seeds of 1 pomegranate (see Tip)

½ cup pecan halves

¼ cup crumbled feta cheese

¼ cup Red Wine Vinaigrette (page 201)

Winter Pear, Beet, and Pomegranate Salad

GRAIN-FREE

Having a wide variety of salads and sides to pull from helps make mealtimes come together with ease. This wintery blend of crisp pear, crunchy pomegranate seeds, pecans, and sweet beets is perfect to lift any cold-weather blues. Bright and packed with flavor, this salad makes a great side dish or a light meal for two. **SERVES 4**

1. In a large saucepan over high heat, cover the beets with water and bring to a boil. Reduce the heat and simmer for 20 to 25 minutes, until the beets are tender when pierced with a fork. Remove from the heat, drain, and set them aside to cool.

2. In a bowl, combine the salad greens, pear slices, pomegranate seeds, pecans, and feta cheese. Toss to combine.

3. Once cooled, peel the beets and thinly slice them. Add them to the salad. Drizzle with the vinaigrette, toss, and serve.

INGREDIENT TIP To remove the seeds from a pomegranate, quarter the fruit and submerge the pieces in a bowl of water. Use your fingers to extract the seeds (which will sink) from the white membrane (which will float). Be sure to protect your clothing while doing this, as pomegranate juice stains.

Per Serving: Calories: 276; Protein: 5g; Cholesterol: 8mg; Sodium: 245mg; Total Carbohydrates: 20g; Fiber: 6g; Total Fat: 21g; Saturated Fat: 4g

Egg *and* Beet Spinach Salad

DAIRY-FREE | GRAIN-FREE | NUT-FREE

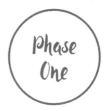

Phase One

PREP TIME: 10 MINUTES
COOK TIME: 25 MINUTES

1 small beet

1 egg

4 cups baby spinach

4 ounces fresh green beans, trimmed

4 tablespoons Red Wine Vinaigrette (page 201)

½ cup sliced radishes

The sweetness of beets and the crunch of fresh green beans are on full display in this salad, which works as a light meal or hearty side dish. If you like loosely set yolks, be sure to run the eggs under cold water to stop the cooking at about 7 minutes. When just right, the creamy yolk blends with the dressing for an amazing combination. **SERVES 2**

1. In a small saucepan, cover the beet and egg with water. Bring to a boil, reduce the heat, and simmer. Remove the egg at 7 minutes for a slightly runny yolk or up to 10 minutes for a firmly cooked one, and run it under cold water to stop the cooking. Continue cooking the beet for a total of 15 to 25 minutes, depending on the size of the beet, until it can be easily pieced with a knife.

2. Peel the egg and cut it into wedges.

3. Run the beet under cool water and use your fingers to remove the skin. Slice the beet thinly.

4. In a large bowl, toss the spinach and green beans. Toss with the Red Wine Vinaigrette and divide the salad into two bowls. Top with the beets, egg, and radishes. Serve.

Per Serving: Calories: 256; Protein: 7g; Cholesterol: 103mg; Sodium: 304mg; Total Carbohydrates: 9g; Fiber: 5g; Total Fat: 21g; Saturated Fat: 3g

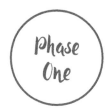

PREP TIME: 15 MINUTES
COOK TIME: 30 MINUTES

¼ cup French green lentils, picked over and rinsed

1 tablespoon canola oil

8 ounces firm tofu, pressed with a towel to remove water, cubed

¼ teaspoon salt, plus more for seasoning

1 tablespoon tamari (see Tip)

3 tablespoons rice vinegar, divided

4 cups salad greens

1 (1-inch) piece fresh ginger, minced

1 teaspoon sesame oil

2 tablespoons extra-virgin olive oil

Freshly ground black pepper

Tofu and Lentil Salad

DAIRY-FREE | GRAIN-FREE | NUT-FREE | VEGAN

A mixture of salad greens, tofu, and lentils creates a protein-rich, hearty meal for two, or a filling side dish for four. French green lentils, which hold their shape well when cooked, are ideal here, but if you don't have them on hand, brown or green lentils will also work; just be sure to remove them from the heat and drain them when they are still al dente so that they retain their shape. SERVES 2 TO 4

1. In a small pot, combine the lentils and 1 cup of water. Bring to a boil over high heat, then reduce the heat and simmer for 15 to 25 minutes, until the lentils are tender. Drain off any excess water.

2. In a large skillet, heat the canola oil over medium-high heat and add the tofu in a single layer. Season lightly with salt. Cook for about 5 minutes, flipping as the tofu browns, until all the sides are lightly browned.

3. Reduce the heat to low and add the tamari and 1 tablespoon of rice vinegar to the skillet. Toss to coat and turn off the heat. Leave to rest in the skillet.

4. Divide the lentils and salad greens between two to four bowls, depending on how many you're serving.

5. In a small bowl, whisk the ginger, sesame oil, olive oil, remaining 2 tablespoons of rice vinegar, 1/4 teaspoon of salt, and pepper. Drizzle over the salad greens and toss to coat. Top with the tofu and serve.

INGREDIENT TIP Tamari is an alternative to traditional soy sauce that minimizes the use of wheat in its production. Made as a by-product of miso fermentation, tamari is a great product to use on a wheat-free diet, although make sure the bottle specifically says that it is gluten-free, as some brands use small amounts of wheat during production. Tamari typically has less sodium than soy sauce, and low-sodium varieties are also available to further cut sodium intake.

Per Serving: Calories: 381; Protein: 17g; Cholesterol: 0mg; Sodium: 824mg; Total Carbohydrates: 19g; Fiber: 9g; Total Fat: 28g; Saturated Fat: 4g

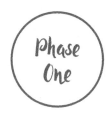

Phase One

PREP TIME: 10 MINUTES
COOK TIME: 5 MINUTES

1 pound broccoli florets, cut into 1-inch pieces

¼ cup red wine vinegar

2 tablespoons whole-grain mustard

2 tablespoons extra-virgin olive oil

2 garlic cloves, minced

½ teaspoon salt

¼ teaspoon freshly ground black pepper

½ cup kalamata olives, halved

½ cup crumbled feta cheese

Broccoli and Olive Salad

GRAIN-FREE | NUT-FREE | UNDER 30 MINUTES

The broccoli in this salad is still slightly crisp, allowing it to hold up well when prepared a day or two in advance. This works great as a side at lunch or dinner, and it can also make a satisfying midday snack. SERVES 4

1. Set a steamer basket over a large pot of boiling water and steam the broccoli for 3 to 5 minutes (making sure the water does not touch the vegetables), until barely fork-tender and still bright green. Remove the broccoli and transfer it to a mixing bowl.

2. In a small bowl, whisk the vinegar, mustard, olive oil, garlic, salt, and pepper. Pour over the broccoli and toss to mix.

3. Add the olives and feta and toss to combine. Serve warm, or refrigerate to serve cold later. The salad can be stored in an airtight container in the refrigerator for up to three days.

Per Serving: Calories: 140; Protein: 10g; Cholesterol: 11mg; Sodium: 483mg; Total Carbohydrates: 7g; Fiber: 2g; Total Fat: 10g; Saturated Fat: 3g

Simple Loaded Coleslaw

DAIRY-FREE | GRAIN-FREE | NUT-FREE | VEGAN

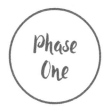

If you think of coleslaw as only shredded cabbage coated in mayo, think again. This delicious slaw uses apple cider vinegar and olive oil to create a tangy dressing that coats the trifecta of cabbage, carrots, and rutabaga in a palate-pleasing way. **SERVES 4**

1. In a food processor with the shredding blade affixed, shred the cabbage, rutabaga, carrots, onion, jalapeño, and garlic. Transfer the vegetables to a large bowl and toss to combine.

2. In a small bowl, mix the apple cider vinegar, salt, pepper, and mustard. Pour over the cabbage mixture and toss to combine. Let the salad rest at room temperature for 30 minutes. Toss to combine right before serving. Refrigerate in an airtight container for up to 3 days.

Per Serving: Calories: 64; Protein: 2g; Cholesterol: 0mg; Sodium: 666mg; Total Carbohydrates: 14g; Fiber: 5g; Total Fat: 0g; Saturated Fat: 0g

PREP TIME: 10 MINUTES, PLUS 30 MINUTES TO REST

½ small red cabbage

1 small rutabaga

2 carrots, trimmed

½ medium red onion

1 small jalapeño pepper, stemmed and seeded

2 garlic cloves

¼ cup apple cider vinegar

½ teaspoon salt

½ teaspoon freshly ground black pepper

1 tablespoon whole-grain mustard

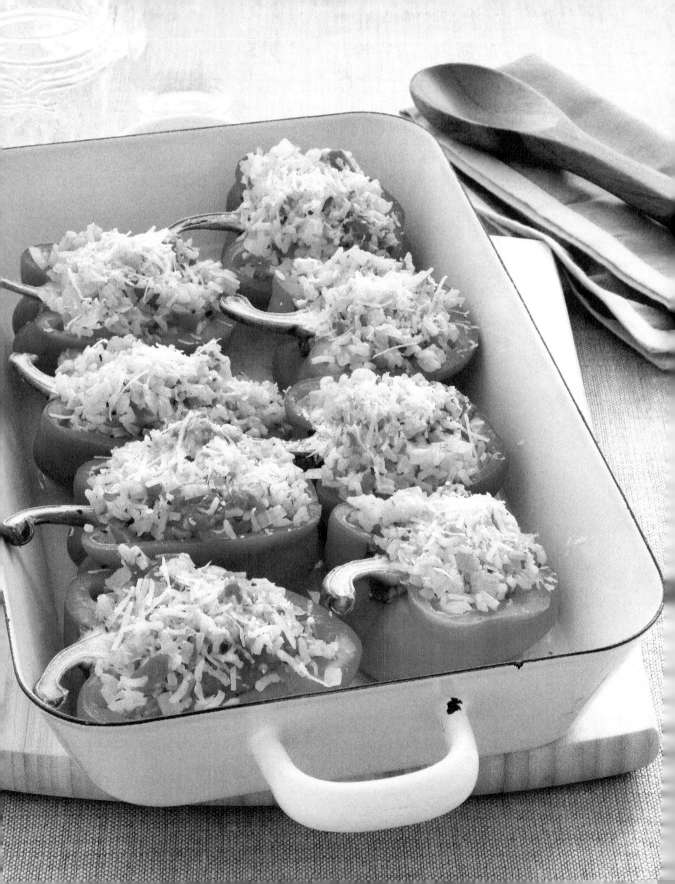

Vegetarian Mains

Vegetables are the cornerstone of the microbiome diet, and these vegetarian main dishes provide tons of fiber while satisfying your taste buds. Covering a wide range of grain and vegetable bowls, as well as hot entrées, this section is where you are able to really dig in and enjoy the bounty of nature.

Arugula and Walnut Quinoa Bowl

UNDER 30 MINUTES

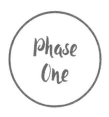

Phase One

Arugula adds a spicy bite to this simple quinoa bowl that you can throw together in a matter of minutes. Be sure to plan ahead and make a large batch of quinoa or other grains to have on hand during the week to use in quick lunch recipes like this one. **SERVES 2**

1. Split the quinoa between two large serving bowls. Top each with 2 cups of arugula, 2 tablespoons of walnuts, 1 tablespoon of flaxseed, and 2 tablespoons of feta.

2. In a small bowl, combine the vinegar and olive oil. Season with the salt and pepper. Divide the dressing between the two bowls and stir well to combine with the quinoa. Serve.

Per Serving: Calories: 381; Protein: 12g; Cholesterol: 17mg; Sodium: 520mg; Total Carbohydrates: 27g; Fiber: 7g; Total Fat: 27g; Saturated Fat: 5g

PREP TIME: 5 MINUTES

1 cup cooked quinoa

4 cups arugula leaves

4 tablespoons walnut pieces

2 tablespoons flaxseed

4 tablespoons crumbled feta cheese

3 tablespoons white wine vinegar

1 tablespoon extra-virgin olive oil

¼ teaspoon salt

¼ teaspoon freshly ground black pepper

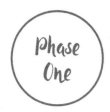

PREP TIME: 10 MINUTES
COOK TIME: 30 MINUTES

1 large spaghetti squash, halved and seeded
1 recipe Tomato Marinara (page 198)
½ cup fresh basil leaves, roughly torn
½ teaspoon salt
¼ cup grated Parmesan cheese

Marinara Spaghetti Squash Noodles

GRAIN-FREE | NUT-FREE

If you are a pasta lover, giving it up can be difficult. While spaghetti squash is not going to trick anyone into believing it's actual pasta, it is a wonderful gluten-free stand-in that delivers. When paired with a classic marinara sauce, it can be an equally satisfying, but microbiome-friendly, comfort food. SERVES 2

1. Preheat the oven to 400°F.

2. Place the squash cut-side down, on a baking sheet. Roast for 30 minutes, until the flesh is tender when pierced with a fork.

3. Meanwhile, in a saucepan, combine the Tomato Marinara and basil, and simmer for 10 minutes.

4. Use a fork to shred the squash into strands and transfer them into the sauce. Stir well and season with the salt.

5. Transfer to two plates, top each with 2 tablespoons of cheese, and serve.

MAKE AHEAD Squash can be roasted up to two days in advance. When cooked, shred the squash and transfer to an airtight container. Let it cool on the counter with the lid off, then cover and refrigerate. When ready to serve, lightly toss the squash in a skillet with a teaspoon of olive oil until heated through and top with marinara and Parmesan.

Per Serving: Calories: 168; Protein: 8g; Cholesterol: 11mg; Sodium: 368mg; Total Carbohydrates: 19g; Fiber: 5g; Total Fat: 8g; Saturated Fat: 8g

Pesto Zucchini Noodles
with Tomatoes

DAIRY-FREE | GRAIN-FREE | VEGAN

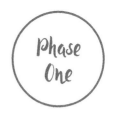

Phase One

Zucchini noodles are a great substitute for pasta, and they are inexpensive to make. If you have a spiralizer, making them is a breeze. If not, a mandolin is a good stand-in. Tossed with a creamy walnut pesto, this pseudo-pasta dish is great either hot or cold. SERVES 4

PREP TIME: 20 MINUTES, PLUS 30 MINUTES TO REST
COOK TIME: 5 MINUTES

TO MAKE THE PESTO

In a blender, process the basil, walnuts, garlic, olive oil, and salt until smooth. If needed, add a little more oil to make the pesto smoother. It should be thick and spreadable. Set it aside.

TO MAKE THE ZUCCHINI NOODLES

1. Using a mandolin, process the zucchini into julienned strips. If you have a julienne blade for your mandolin, use that. If not, slice it lengthwise on the mandolin and then use a knife to cut it into thin strips.

2. Transfer the zucchini strips to a colander and toss with the salt. Let them rest over the sink for 30 minutes. Lightly press the zucchini to extract as much liquid as possible.

3. In a large skillet, heat the olive oil over medium heat. Add the zucchini and toss for 2 to 3 minutes. until just heated through. Add the tomatoes and toss for 1 minute more. Stir in the pesto until combined and serve.

Per Serving: Calories: 352; Protein: 8g; Cholesterol: 0mg; Sodium: 593mg; Total Carbohydrates: 18g; Fiber: 6g; Total Fat: 31g; Saturated Fat: 4g

FOR THE PESTO
2 cups fresh basil leaves
½ cup walnut pieces
3 garlic cloves
⅓ cup extra-virgin olive oil
½ teaspoon salt

FOR THE ZUCCHINI NOODLES
8 medium zucchini, peeled
½ teaspoon salt
2 teaspoons extra-virgin olive oil
2 small tomatoes, diced

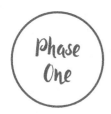

PREP TIME: 10 MINUTES
COOK TIME: 40 MINUTES

½ cup millet

2 teaspoons extra-virgin olive oil, plus more for oiling the peppers

4 red bell peppers, halved, seeded, and cored

1 small red onion, diced

2 garlic cloves, minced

1 small tomato, diced

½ teaspoon salt

¼ teaspoon freshly ground black pepper

1 (15-ounce) can low-sodium chickpeas

½ cup shredded Parmesan cheese

Mediterranean Millet-Stuffed Peppers

NUT-FREE

Millet is one of the earliest cultivated cereal grains and a perfect stand-in for wheat if you're on a gluten-free diet. It cooks quickly, is rich in B vitamins, and is one of the easiest grains to digest. Because millet can spoil more quickly than other grains, be sure to purchase it in small quantities and store it in a cool location. For an eye-catching presentation on the table, leave the bell pepper stems intact and just remove the inner cores. SERVES 4

1. Preheat the oven to 350°F.

2. In a small saucepan, combine the millet and 1¼ water. Bring to a boil over medium-high heat, reduce the heat, cover, and simmer for 10 to 15 minutes, until all the water has been absorbed. Let the millet stand for 10 minutes.

3. Lightly oil the skins of the peppers and place them on a baking sheet with the cavities facing up.

4. In a large skillet, heat the remaining 2 teaspoons of olive oil over medium-high heat. Add the onion and cook for 3 to 5 minutes, stirring regularly, until it softens. Add the garlic and cook for 1 minute more. Add the tomato and stir for 1 minute, until heated through.

5. Stir in the cooked millet and season with the salt and pepper. Add the chickpeas and mix well.

6. Scoop the millet mixture into the prepared peppers and top with the Parmesan cheese. Cover with aluminum foil and bake for 15 minutes, until heated through and the cheese has melted. If desired, broil for 3 to 5 minutes to brown the tops. Serve.

Per Serving: Calories: 295; Protein: 13g; Cholesterol: 7mg; Sodium: 603mg; Total Carbohydrates: 43g; Fiber: 9g; Total Fat: 8g; Saturated Fat: 3g

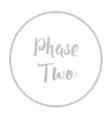

PREP TIME: 10 MINUTES
COOK TIME: 35 MINUTES

2 medium eggplants,
   sliced lengthwise

1 teaspoon extra-virgin
   olive oil

1 medium yellow
   onion, diced

3 garlic cloves, minced

2 carrots, shredded

2 cups cooked brown rice
   (see page 81)

¼ cup golden raisins

1 (15-ounce) can chickpeas

2 tablespoons chopped
   fresh mint leaves

2 tablespoons chopped
   fresh parsley leaves

2 tablespoons freshly
   squeezed lemon juice

¼ teaspoon
   ground cinnamon

½ teaspoon salt

Brown Rice–Stuffed Eggplant

DAIRY-FREE | NUT-FREE | VEGAN

Eggplant takes on pretty much any flavor you offer it. Which is good, because this rice stuffing brings plenty of flavor! Whip up a Simple Green Side Salad (page 107) or a crisp Fragrant Fennel and Kohlrabi Salad (page 109) while the eggplant cooks, and dinner is served. SERVES 4

1. In a large skillet, place the eggplants cut-side down and add about 1 inch of water. Place the skillet over medium-high heat and bring the water to a boil. Simmer for 10 minutes, until the eggplant flesh is tender.

2. Remove the eggplants from the skillet and let sit until they are cool to the touch. Scoop out and reserve the flesh, leaving about a ½-inch shell. Arrange the shells on a baking sheet with the cavity facing up.

3. Preheat the oven to 350°F.

4. In the wiped-out skillet, heat the olive oil and add the reserved eggplant, onion, and garlic, cooking for 5 minutes, stirring frequently, until the onion begins to soften. Add the carrots, rice, raisins, and chickpeas. Stir well and continue to cook for 5 minutes.

5. Stir in the mint, parsley, lemon juice, cinnamon, and salt. Spoon the mixture into the shells and bake for 20 minutes, until lightly browned. Serve.

MAKE AHEAD Cook the eggplant, prepare the stuffing, and stuff the eggplant the night before. Store, covered, in the refrigerator until ready to bake; increase the cooking time by 5 minutes.

Per Serving: Calories: 332; Protein: 11g; Cholesterol: 0mg; Sodium: 461mg; Total Carbohydrates: 68g; Fiber: 17g; Total Fat: 4g; Saturated Fat: 1g

Italian Lentil Salad

DAIRY-FREE | GRAIN-FREE | NUT-FREE | VEGAN

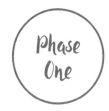

Phase One

This hearty lentil salad has plenty of flavor, much of it imparted from the olives and tomatoes that season it so wonderfully. Make it the night before to allow the flavors to meld before serving. **SERVES 4**

PREP TIME: 10 MINUTES
COOK TIME: 25 MINUTES, PLUS 30 MINUTES TO CHILL

1. In a small saucepan, combine the lentils and 3 cups of water. Bring to a boil over high heat, reduce the heat to medium, and cook for 15 to 25 minutes, until the lentils are just tender. Drain and rinse them under cool water.

2. In a large bowl, toss the scallions, tomatoes, cucumber, and olives. Add the lentils and toss gently. Add the olive oil, lemon juice, and salt. Stir to combine. Refrigerate for at least 30 minutes and stir before serving.

1 cup French green lentils, picked through and rinsed

6 scallions, white and green parts, thinly sliced

1 cup chopped tomatoes

1 cucumber, peeled and diced

¼ cup pitted kalamata olives, sliced

3 tablespoons extra-virgin olive oil

¼ cup freshly squeezed lemon juice

½ teaspoon salt

Per Serving: Calories: 307; Protein: 14g; Cholesterol: 0mg; Sodium: 429mg; Total Carbohydrates: 35g; Fiber: 16g; Total Fat: 13g; Saturated Fat: 2g

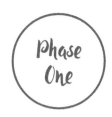

Phase One

PREP TIME: 10 MINUTES
COOK TIME: 25 MINUTES

1 cup French green lentils, picked through and rinsed (see Tip)

3 cups low-sodium vegetable broth

1 large carrot, finely diced

2 celery stalks, finely diced

2 garlic cloves, minced

1 teaspoon whole-grain mustard

2 tablespoons freshly squeezed lemon juice

2 tablespoons extra-virgin olive oil

½ teaspoon salt

¼ teaspoon freshly ground black pepper

¼ cup crumbled goat cheese

Goat Cheese *and* Lentil Salad

GRAIN-FREE | NUT-FREE

Lentils are not all the same, and seeking out a few different varieties can make the difference between love and hate of this legume. For lentil salads, use French green lentils, which hold their shape well after cooking. Unlike lettuce salads, lentil salads are actually best when made in advance so the flavors have time to mingle. Refrigerate this salad for at least a couple of hours before serving, if possible. Bring to room temperature before serving and adjust the seasoning as needed. **SERVES 4**

1. In a large saucepan, combine the lentils and broth and bring to a boil over high heat. Reduce the heat and simmer for 15 to 25 minutes, until the lentils are tender. Drain the lentils of any remaining broth and let them cool.

2. In a large bowl, mix the carrot, celery, and garlic. Add the lentils and toss to combine.

3. In a small bowl, combine the mustard, lemon juice, and olive oil. Season with the salt and pepper. Pour the dressing over the lentils and toss gently to coat. Divide between two plates and top with the goat cheese. Serve.

INGREDIENT TIP Brown lentils, the type most commonly sold in stores, work best in soups and stuffing, where maintaining their shape is not critical. When fully cooked, these lentils tend to fall apart, which is a consistency that works great in curries, soups, and stuffing, but not as well in salads.

Per Serving: Calories: 283; Protein: 14g; Cholesterol: 5mg; Sodium: 485mg; Total Carbohydrates: 35g; Fiber: 17g; Total Fat: 9g; Saturated Fat: 2g

Moroccan Date and Carrot Lentil Salad

DAIRY-FREE | GRAIN-FREE | NUT-FREE | VEGAN

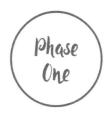

PREP TIME: 10 MINUTES
COOK TIME: 35 MINUTES

While this dish is traditionally made using preserved lemon, this quick and easy version uses a lemon-garlic vinaigrette that you can whip up at home in a few minutes. Like other lentil salads, this one benefits from chilling in the refrigerator for at least 2 hours before serving. Served hot or cold, this lentil dish is great for both lunch and dinner. SERVES 4

1 cup French green lentils, picked through and rinsed

½ teaspoon salt

1 tablespoon extra-virgin olive oil

1 cup diced carrot

1 cup diced yellow onion

6 dates, pitted and thinly sliced

¼ cup sliced fresh mint leaves

¼ cup Bright Lemon-Garlic Vinaigrette (page 202)

1. In a large saucepan, combine the lentils and 3 cups of water. Bring to a boil over high heat, reduce the heat to medium-low, and simmer for 10 minutes. Add the salt and continue to cook until the lentils are just tender, another 5 to 15 minutes. Drain well.

2. In a large skillet, heat the olive oil over medium heat. Add the carrot and onion, and cook for about 10 minutes, until tender. Remove from the heat.

3. Add the lentils and dates to the skillet and toss well. Stir in the mint. Add the vinaigrette and to stir to combine thoroughly. Serve.

MAKE AHEAD Make and refrigerate, covered, for up to 2 days, but hold off on adding the mint until you are ready to serve the dish.

Per Serving: Calories: 323; Protein: 14g; Cholesterol: 0mg; Sodium: 463mg; Total Carbohydrates: 45g; Fiber: 17g; Total Fat: 11g; Saturated Fat: 2g

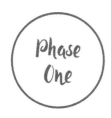

PREP TIME: 10 MINUTES
COOK TIME: 45 MINUTES

½ cup green or brown lentils, picked through and rinsed

4 medium zucchini, cut lengthwise (see Tip)

1 tablespoon extra-virgin olive oil

1 shallot, diced

2 garlic cloves, minced

3 cups roughly chopped baby spinach

1 cup Tomato Marinara (page 198)

¼ teaspoon red pepper flakes

½ cup shredded mozzarella cheese

Lentil-Stuffed Zucchini

GRAIN-FREE | NUT-FREE

Lentils make a great vegetarian protein because they are so meaty and dense. Fill these little squash boats (for how to make them, see Tip), and you won't miss the meat in this satiating meal. SERVES 4

1. In a small saucepan, combine the lentils and 2 cups of water. Bring to a boil over high heat, reduce the heat, and simmer for 15 minutes, until the lentils are just tender. Drain the lentils and run them under cold water to stop the cooking.

2. Preheat the oven to 400°F.

3. Use a firm teaspoon to dig out the seeds from the zucchini, and scrape out enough flesh so that only a ¼-inch border remains around the whole zucchini. Roughly chop the flesh into small pieces. Transfer the zucchini boats to a large baking dish with the cavities facing up.

4. In a large skillet, heat the olive oil over medium-high heat. Add the shallot and cook for 3 minutes, until it begins to brown. Add the garlic and cook for 1 minute more, stirring constantly. Add the zucchini flesh and cook for 2 to 3 minutes, until softened.

5. Add the spinach, stirring until it wilts. Pour the marinara into the skillet and stir to coat. Add the red pepper flakes and lentils to the pan and cook for 2 minutes more.

6. Divide the mixture evenly between the prepared zucchini and top with the mozzarella. Cover with aluminum foil and bake for 30 minutes.

7. Remove the foil and transfer to the broiler for 3 to 5 minutes to brown the tops. Serve.

INGREDIENT TIP Try to find plump, wide-bottomed zucchini, which makes stuffing them all the easier.

Per Serving: Calories: 262; Protein: 17g; Cholesterol: 19mg; Sodium: 281mg; Total Carbohydrates: 28g; Fiber: 11g; Total Fat: 11g; Saturated Fat: 4g

Black Bean *and* Quinoa Bowl

DAIRY-FREE | NUT-FREE | VEGAN | UNDER 30 MINUTES

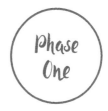

Phase One

Showing yet another use of versatile quinoa, this bowl features black beans and a lime vinaigrette that gives it its Southwestern flair. Depending on your mood, serve this hot or cold, and if you are in phase two of the microbiome diet, considering adding a scant handful of diced chicken on top for a little more protein. **SERVES 4**

1. Into each of four bowls, put ½ cup of quinoa. Top each with ½ cup of black beans, and one-fourth of the red pepper, tomato, and scallions.

2. In a small bowl, whisk together the olive oil, cumin, garlic powder, lime juice, and salt. Drizzle the dressing over the bowls and serve.

Per Serving: Calories: 402; Protein: 19g; Cholesterol: 0mg; Sodium: 614mg; Total Carbohydrates: 63g; Fiber: 20g; Total Fat: 9g; Saturated Fat: 1g

PREP TIME: 10 MINUTES

2 cups cooked quinoa

2 (15-ounce) cans low-sodium black beans, rinsed and drained

1 red bell pepper, seeded and diced

1 tomato, diced

1 bunch scallions, white and green parts, chopped

2 tablespoons extra-virgin olive oil

1 teaspoon ground cumin

½ teaspoon garlic powder

Juice of 2 limes

½ teaspoon salt

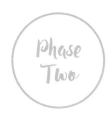

Phase Two

PREP TIME: 10 MINUTES
COOK TIME: 5 MINUTES

2 (15-ounce) cans
low-sodium black beans,
rinsed and drained

2 teaspoons Taco
Seasoning (page 197)

2 cups cooked brown rice
(see page 81)

2 cups salad greens

1 cup Fermented
Salsa (page 217) or
store-bought salsa

1 avocado, diced

¼ cup chopped
fresh cilantro

Black Bean Burrito Bowl

DAIRY-FREE | NUT-FREE | VEGAN | UNDER 30 MINUTES

This filling meal has all the trimmings of a burrito, just without the tortilla. You won't miss a thing though, as the flavor of the beans, salsa, avocado, and cilantro ties the whole bowl together so well. If desired, add a sprinkling of shredded cheese. SERVES 4

1. In a small saucepan, combine the beans and 1 cup of water. Bring to a boil over high heat, then reduce the heat and add the Taco Seasoning. Simmer for 2 to 3 minutes, until heated through.

2. Into each of four bowls, put ½ cup of rice. Top with one-fourth of the black beans, a handful of salad greens, ¼ cup of salsa, several avocado pieces, and 1 tablespoon of cilantro. Serve.

Per Serving: Calories: 409; Protein: 18g; Cholesterol: 0mg; Sodium: 351mg; Total Carbohydrates: 68g; Fiber: 21g; Total Fat: 9g; Saturated Fat: 1g

Black Bean Veggie Burgers

DAIRY-FREE | GRAIN-FREE | UNDER 30 MINUTES

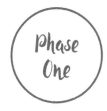

Black beans are so versatile that it is possible for them to star in many recipes in your diet. As a burger, they are meaty and creamy, forming into a patty perfectly. Serve these flavorful burgers on a bed of Cauliflower Rice (page 188), or opt for the deconstructed lettuce-wrapped burger laid out here. **SERVES 4**

PREP TIME: 10 MINUTES
COOK TIME: 10 MINUTES

2 (15-ounce) cans low-sodium black beans, rinsed and drained

1 teaspoon garlic powder

1 teaspoon onion powder

¼ teaspoon cayenne pepper

1 cup almond flour

¼ cup grated yellow onion

1 egg

2 teaspoons extra-virgin olive oil

4 large lettuce leaves

1 tomato, sliced, for serving

Ketchup (page 199), or store-bought, for serving

Mustard, for serving

1. In a large bowl, mash the beans well with a fork, leaving a few bean pieces here and there. Mix in the garlic powder, onion powder, cayenne, almond flour, onion, and egg. Stir well to combine.

2. In a large skillet, heat the olive oil over medium-high heat.

3. Form the bean mixture into four patties and place them in the skillet. Cook on one side for 3 to 5 minutes, until browned. Flip and continue to cook on the other side for 3 minutes more.

4. Place the burgers on the lettuce leaves, top with tomato slices, Ketchup, and mustard, and wrap the leaf around the burger to serve.

Per Serving: Calories: 580; Protein: 28g; Cholesterol: 52mg; Sodium: 332mg; Total Carbohydrates: 52g; Fiber: 22g; Total Fat: 33g; Saturated Fat: 3g

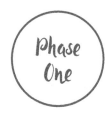

Phase One

PREP TIME: 5 MINUTES
COOK TIME: 25 MINUTES

1 cup buckwheat groats
(see Tip)

4 scallions, white and
green parts, thinly sliced

1 bunch parsley,
finely chopped

¼ cup finely chopped fresh
mint leaves

Juice of 1 lemon

2 tablespoons extra-virgin
olive oil

½ teaspoon salt

¼ teaspoon freshly ground
black pepper

1 cup sliced radishes

1 (15-ounce) can chickpeas,
rinsed and drained

1 avocado, sliced lengthwise

Chickpea and Avocado Buckwheat Tabbouleh

DAIRY-FREE | NUT-FREE | VEGAN

Though its name indicates otherwise, buckwheat does not actually contain any wheat. This lesser-known grain is an interesting stand-in for bulgur in this microbiome-friendly tabbouleh. Tossed with chickpeas, avocado, and radishes, this multitextured dish makes a filling lunch or dinner. Be sure to keep an eye on the buckwheat to prevent it from overcooking and becoming mushy. SERVES 4

1. Heat a medium saucepan over medium-high heat. Add the groats and toast, stirring constantly, for 5 minutes, until browned and toasted.

2. Add 2 cups of water and bring to a boil. Reduce the heat to low and simmer for 15 to 20 minutes, until the groats are just tender. Drain them in a colander and rinse gently under cold water to stop the cooking. Leave them to drain over the sink.

3. In a large bowl, mix the scallions, parsley, and mint. Stir in the buckwheat. Add the lemon juice, olive oil, salt, and pepper. Toss to combine.

4. Divide the tabbouleh between four bowls and top each with ¼ cup of radishes, scant ½ cup of chickpeas, and 3 or 4 avocado slices. Serve.

INGREDIENT TIP Find buckwheat groats at health food stores or a well-stocked grocery store with a bulk-food section. If you like the flavor, try making a hot cereal from ground buckwheat. It is a tasty gluten-free porridge that goes well with nuts and dried fruits for a filling breakfast.

Per Serving: Calories: 387; Protein: 11g; Cholesterol: 0mg; Sodium: 456mg; Total Carbohydrates: 53g; Fiber: 13g; Total Fat: 17g; Saturated Fat: 2g

Chickpea and Spinach Stir-Fry

DAIRY-FREE | GRAIN-FREE | VEGAN | UNDER 30 MINUTES

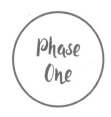

PREP TIME: 10 MINUTES
COOK TIME: 15 MINUTES

Chickpeas are firmer than many other beans, making them a perfect star in a meatless stir-fry. Mixed with warming garlic, red pepper flakes, and cumin, this is a lovely and super-fast one-pan dish that the whole family will enjoy. SERVES 4 TO 6

1 tablespoon extra-virgin olive oil

1 large yellow onion, diced

4 garlic cloves, minced

1 tablespoon ground cumin

½ teaspoon salt

1 large tomato, diced

2 (15-ounce) cans low-sodium chickpeas, rinsed and drained

1½ cups baby spinach

Freshly ground black pepper

Red pepper flakes

1. In a large skillet, heat the olive oil over medium-high heat, and sauté the onion for 3 to 5 minutes, until it begins to brown. Add the garlic to the skillet and cook for 1 minute, until just fragrant.

2. Add the cumin and toss to coat. Stir constantly for 1 minute and then add the salt, tomato, chickpeas, and 1 cup of water. Simmer for 5 minutes.

3. Stir in the spinach in batches, adding more as the spinach wilts, until it has all been incorporated. Season with freshly ground black pepper and red pepper flakes, and serve.

DID YOU KNOW? Canned beans have a lot of salt already added, so don't be too heavy-handed with the salt when using them. Look for low-sodium versions, which minimize your sodium intake but still are robustly salty. Much of that sodium is contained in the cooking liquid, so be sure to drain canned beans well and rinse them with water before using.

Per Serving: Calories: 249; Protein: 12g; Cholesterol: 0mg; Sodium: 629mg; Total Carbohydrates: 37g; Fiber: 11g; Total Fat: 7g; Saturated Fat: 1g

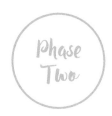

PREP TIME: 10 MINUTES
COOK TIME: 5 MINUTES

FOR THE SAUCE

2 tablespoons tamari

2 tablespoons rice vinegar

1 tablespoon honey

**FOR THE KUNG PAO
CHICKPEAS**

1 tablespoon canola oil

2 (15-ounce) cans
chickpeas, rinsed
and drained

4 garlic cloves, minced

1 (1-inch) piece fresh
ginger, minced

1 teaspoon red
pepper flakes

4 scallions, white and
green parts, thinly sliced

½ cup unsalted peanuts

2 teaspoons sesame oil

Kung Pao Chickpeas

DAIRY-FREE | GRAIN-FREE | UNDER 30 MINUTES

Using honey to impart its classic sweetness, this kung pao dish is revamped to fuel the microbiome. Even though it is vegetarian, because it does use a sweetener, it needs to be reserved for phase two of the diet. SERVES 4

TO MAKE THE SAUCE

In a small bowl, mix the tamari, rice vinegar, and honey. Set it aside.

TO MAKE THE KUNG PAO CHICKPEAS

1. In a large skillet, heat the canola oil over medium heat. Add the chickpeas and stir for 2 to 3 minutes, until they begin to brown. Add the garlic, ginger, red pepper flakes, and scallions, and stir for 1 minute more.

2. Give the sauce a stir and add it to the skillet. Cook for 1 minute, stirring constantly until thickened. Add the peanuts and sesame oil, toss to combine, and serve.

DID YOU KNOW? Most store-bought sauces contain sweeteners and fillers to enhance their flavor, texture, and shelf life. For this reason, it is important to make your own sauces, such as this one, at home. If desired, you can mix this sauce up to a day in advance to speed up mealtime on a busy night.

Per Serving: Calories: 365; Protein: 15g; Cholesterol: 0mg; Sodium: 777mg; Total Carbohydrates: 40g; Fiber: 10g; Total Fat: 18g; Saturated Fat: 2g

Malaysian-Style Coconut Tofu and Vegetable Curry

DAIRY-FREE | GRAIN-FREE | NUT-FREE | UNDER 30 MINUTES

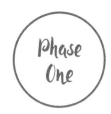

Phase One

Malaysian curry is a rich coconut-milk treat, teeming with savory ginger, lemongrass, and chile flavors. Once you have the paste made, all the heavy lifting is complete. Fry it gently and combine it with the coconut milk for a sumptuous meal. Serve over Cauliflower Rice (page 188) for a completely satisfying vegetable-forward dinner. SERVES 4

PREP TIME: 10 MINUTES
COOK TIME: 15 MINUTES

FOR THE CURRY PASTE

1 (1-inch) piece fresh ginger

1 lemongrass stalk, outer layers, root, and woody top parts removed

1 fresh red chile, stemmed and seeded

1 red onion, diced

2 garlic cloves, chopped

1 teaspoon ground turmeric

¼ teaspoon salt

1 tablespoon coconut oil

FOR THE CURRY

1 (15-ounce) can light coconut milk

1 cup low-sodium vegetable broth

8 ounces fresh snow peas or snap peas

1½ tablespoons coconut oil, divided

1 (12-ounce) package firm tofu, cubed and patted dry (see Tip)

8 ounces cremini mushrooms

TO MAKE THE CURRY PASTE

Place the ginger, lemongrass, chile, onion, garlic, turmeric, salt, and coconut oil in a blender and process until smooth.

TO MAKE THE CURRY

1. Heat a large skillet over medium-high heat and cook the curry paste for 2 minutes, stirring constantly, until fragrant. Add the coconut milk and broth, and stir to combine. Bring to a simmer and then reduce the heat to medium. Add the peas and simmer for 5 minutes, and then remove from the heat.

2. In a small skillet, heat 1 tablespoon of coconut oil over medium-high heat. Add the tofu cubes and cook for 3 to 5 minutes, stirring regularly, until lightly browned on all sides. Transfer the tofu to the curry.

3. Add the remaining ½ tablespoon of coconut oil to the small skillet and heat over medium-high heat. Sauté the mushrooms for 3 minutes, until softened lightly, and add to the curry. Serve.

INGREDIENT TIP When pan-frying tofu, it is important to first press the tofu well with a paper towel or clean kitchen towel to remove moisture. This will prevent it from sticking to the pan and ensure it gets a nice browned exterior.

Per Serving: Calories: 268; Protein: 11g; Cholesterol: 0mg; Sodium: 195mg; Total Carbohydrates: 14g; Fiber: 3g; Total Fat: 19g; Saturated Fat: 13g

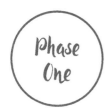

PREP TIME: 10 MINUTES
COOK TIME: 15 MINUTES

2 teaspoons extra-virgin
   olive oil, divided

3 teaspoons tamari, divided

8 ounces firm tofu,
   finely diced

1 (1-inch) piece fresh
   ginger, minced

3 garlic cloves, minced

1 carrot, shredded

2 cups chopped
   broccoli florets

1 cup sliced
   cremini mushrooms

1 teaspoon sesame oil

2 tablespoons rice vinegar

4 scallions, white and
   green parts, chopped

1 (7-ounce) package
   shirataki noodles, drained
   and rinsed

1 tablespoon sesame
   seeds, for garnish

Shirataki, Vegetable, and Tofu Stir-Fry

DAIRY-FREE | GRAIN-FREE | NUT-FREE | VEGAN | UNDER 30 MINUTES

This Asian-style stir-fry comes together in minutes yet tastes as though it took much longer. Try pre-chopping your veggies when you have a few extra minutes earlier in the week, and you can get this dish prepared in just 15 minutes. **SERVES 2**

1. In a large skillet, heat 1 teaspoon of olive oil over medium-high heat. Add 1 teaspoon of tamari and the tofu, and cook, stirring constantly, for 5 minutes, until the tofu begins to lightly brown. Transfer to a serving plate.

2. Add the remaining 1 teaspoon of olive oil to the skillet and heat over medium-high heat. Add the ginger and garlic, stirring constantly, for 1 minute. Add the carrot, broccoli florets, and mushrooms. Cook for about 5 minutes, until the broccoli is bright green and the mushrooms have begun to soften.

3. In a small bowl, mix the remaining 2 teaspoons of tamari, the sesame oil, and rice vinegar. Add this sauce, the scallions, shirataki noodles, and cooked tofu to the pan and stir for 5 more minutes, until the sauce thickens and coats the vegetables. Serve topped with the sesame seeds.

Per Serving: Calories: 260; Protein: 17g; Cholesterol: 0mg; Sodium: 588mg; Total Carbohydrates: 21g; Fiber: 8g; Total Fat: 15g; Saturated Fat: 2g

Balsamic Mushroom *and* Corn Stir-Fry

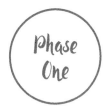

DAIRY-FREE | GRAIN-FREE | NUT-FREE | VEGAN | UNDER 30 MINUTES

Mushrooms have a certain meaty quality that makes them great as a main course. Here in this simple stir-fry, they are elevated with balsamic vinegar, which complements the vegetables with a hit of flavor. **SERVES 4**

PREP TIME: 10 MINUTES
COOK TIME: 10 MINUTES

2 tablespoons extra-virgin olive oil

4 garlic cloves, minced

16 ounces cremini mushrooms, diced

1 bell pepper, stemmed, seeded, and diced

2 cups corn kernels (fresh or frozen and thawed)

3 tablespoons balsamic vinegar

Freshly ground black pepper

1. In a large skillet, heat the olive oil over medium heat. Add the garlic and sauté for 1 minute, until just fragrant. Add the mushrooms and bell pepper, and stir regularly for 3 to 5 minutes, until the mushrooms begin to leave some water in the pan.

2. Add the corn and stir to mix. Cover the skillet and let the vegetables steam for 3 to 5 minutes, until the corn is tender and heated through. Add the balsamic vinegar, season with pepper, and stir. Serve.

MAKE AHEAD The taste of this dish only deepens with a little time spent resting. Make this up to a day in advance, cool, and refrigerate. To reheat, toss it in a heated pan over medium heat until hot, or reheat in the microwave.

Per Serving: Calories: 186; Protein: 7g; Cholesterol: 0mg; Sodium: 14mg; Total Carbohydrates: 28g; Fiber: 4g; Total Fat: 8g; Saturated Fat: 1g

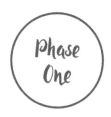

Phase One

PREP TIME: 10 MINUTES
COOK TIME: 20 MINUTES

1 teaspoon extra-virgin olive
  oil, plus 1 tablespoon

1 medium yellow onion,
  finely diced

6 ounces cremini
  mushrooms, finely
  chopped

1 (12-ounce) package
  firm tofu

¼ cup roughly chopped
  basil leaves

4 garlic cloves

¾ cup almond flour, divided

¾ cup flaxseed
  meal, divided

1 egg

2 tablespoons
  balsamic vinegar

4 large lettuce leaves,
  for serving

Ketchup (page 199), or
  store-bought, for serving

Mustard, for serving

Mushroom Tofu Burgers

DAIRY-FREE | GRAIN-FREE

Mushrooms give this tofu burger some serious bulk and bite. A blend of almond flour and flaxseed meal helps solidify the simple burger and give it a firm texture that holds up well. This meat-free burger is filling and loaded with flavor. Wrap it in a large lettuce leaf and top with your favorite condiments. **SERVES 4**

1. In a large skillet, heat 1 teaspoon of olive oil over medium heat. Add the onion and cook until softened, 5 to 7 minutes. Add the mushrooms and cook for another 3 minutes. Turn the heat off and transfer the vegetables to a bowl to cool slightly.

2. In a food processor, combine the tofu, basil, and garlic and process until smooth. Transfer to a mixing bowl.

3. Add the mushroom and onion mixture to the bowl, along with ½ cup of almond flour, ½ cup of flaxseed meal, the egg, and balsamic vinegar.

4. In a small bowl, mix the remaining ¼ cup of almond flour and ¼ cup of flaxseed meal. Form the mushroom mixture into four patties and lightly coat each patty in the flour mixture.

5. In a skillet, heat the remaining 1 tablespoon of olive oil over medium heat. Add the burgers and cook for 3 to 5 minutes on each side, until browned.

6. To serve, wrap each burger in a lettuce leaf and top with Ketchup, mustard, and other favorite condiments.

MAKE AHEAD Burgers are great make-ahead fare. To prepare these in advance, form the patties and coat in almond flour and flaxseed meal. Lay them in a single layer on a baking sheet and freeze for 2 hours. Once frozen solid, transfer them to a freezer-safe storage bag or container and store frozen for up to 1 month. When ready to serve, heat in the oven, on the stove top, or in the toaster oven until heated through and browned.

Per Serving: Calories: 478; Protein: 24g; Cholesterol: 52mg; Sodium: 42mg; Total Carbohydrates: 23g; Fiber: 12g; Total Fat: 36g; Saturated Fat: 4g

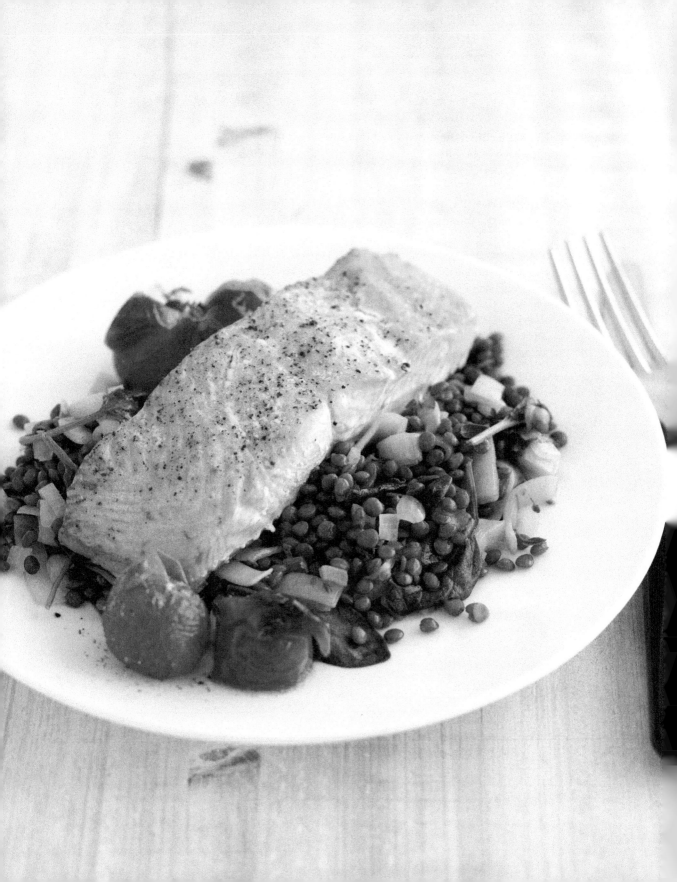

Seafood Mains

While meat is off the table in phase one, you can enjoy fish and seafood. This section includes a wide variety of tasty and healthy meals. These recipes are designed for ease, both in preparation and cooking, and offer mouthwatering flavor that satisfies.

Salmon Salad Lettuce Wraps

GRAIN-FREE | NUT-FREE | UNDER 30 MINUTES

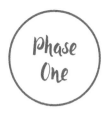

Salmon is a wonderful lunch treat, and when you can get it in a can just like tuna, it is easy and quick. Look for boneless skinless salmon sold in small cans. The larger cans, which contain skin and bones, are great for making patties and other cooked dishes, but for preparations out of the can, the smaller size is best. **SERVES 2**

PREP TIME: 10 MINUTES

1 (6-ounce) can boneless skinless salmon

¼ cup diced celery

¼ cup unsweetened plain yogurt

1 teaspoon freshly squeezed lemon juice

¼ teaspoon salt

2 tablespoons chopped fresh cilantro

8 large lettuce leaves

1. Drain the salmon in a fine-mesh strainer over the sink. Press the salmon with the back of a spoon to expel as much liquid as possible. Transfer it to a small bowl.

2. Add the celery, yogurt, lemon juice, salt, and cilantro and mix well.

3. Arrange the lettuce leaves on two plates and spoon about a tablespoon of the mixture onto each lettuce leaf. Wrap each leaf around the salmon salad and serve.

MAKE AHEAD Mix the salmon salad up to 1 day in advance. Refrigerate in an airtight container and remix before filling the lettuce wraps and serving.

Per Serving: Calories: 207; Protein: 22g; Cholesterol: 3mg; Sodium: 717mg; Total Carbohydrates: 4g; Fiber: 1g; Total Fat: 12g; Saturated Fat: 3g

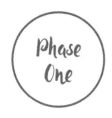

Phase One

PREP TIME: 10 MINUTES

1 (6-ounce) can tuna
packed in water, drained

¼ cup diced celery

¼ cup unsweetened
plain yogurt

1 teaspoon whole-grain
mustard

Freshly ground
black pepper

8 large lettuce leaves

Tuna Salad Lettuce Wraps

GRAIN-FREE | NUT-FREE | UNDER 30 MINUTES

Tuna is a classic lunch favorite. Here it is given a remake with probiotic superstar yogurt in place of the typical mayonnaise. Whip the salad up in minutes and have it on hand for a quick light lunch or dinner that satisfies. Whole-grain mustard gives these wraps an added kick; if you don't have it, try Dijon instead or just leave it out. **SERVES 2**

1. Drain the tuna in a fine-mesh strainer over the sink. Press the tuna with the back of a spoon to expel as much liquid as possible. Transfer it to a small bowl.

2. Add the celery, yogurt, and mustard and season with pepper. Mix well.

3. Arrange the lettuce leaves on two serving plates and spoon about a tablespoon of the mixture onto each lettuce leaf. Wrap each leaf around the tuna salad and serve.

MAKE AHEAD Mix the tuna salad up to 1 day in advance. Refrigerate in an airtight container and remix before filling the lettuce wraps and serving.

SUBSTITUTION TIP For a heartier option, spoon the mixture into a cucumber that has been halved and seeded. The simple veggie shell has a nice crunch that complements the tuna well.

Per Serving: Calories: 143; Protein: 22g; Cholesterol: 40mg; Sodium: 395mg; Total Carbohydrates: 4g; Fiber: 1g; Total Fat: 4g; Saturated Fat: 1g

Simple Roasted
Salmon Fillets with Tomatoes

DAIRY-FREE | GRAIN-FREE | NUT-FREE | UNDER 30 MINUTES

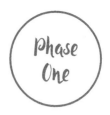

Phase One

PREP TIME: 5 MINUTES
COOK TIME: 15 MINUTES

Salmon is a fish that requires little extra to make it shine. In this simple recipe, fillets are panfried along with cherry tomatoes. The main course comes together with less than 5 minutes of hands-on prep time, giving you a chance to throw together a salad or other simple side while it cooks. If you have extra salmon, separate it into flakes and make it into Salmon Salad (page 145). **SERVES 4**

1 pound salmon fillets

¾ teaspoon salt, divided

½ teaspoon freshly ground black pepper

3 teaspoons extra-virgin olive oil, divided

1 pint cherry tomatoes

1 teaspoon dried dill

1. Season the salmon with ½ teaspoon of salt and the pepper. Set it aside.

2. In a large skillet, heat 1 teaspoon of olive oil over medium heat. Add the tomatoes and the remaining ¼ teaspoon of salt. Sauté the tomatoes for 3 to 5 minutes, until they are heated through and soft. Add the dill and stir to combine. Transfer to a serving dish.

3. In the same skillet, heat the remaining 2 teaspoons of oil over medium heat. Place the salmon, flesh-side down, in the skillet. After 3 minutes, flip the salmon and continue to cook for 5 to 8 minutes more, until the fish is cooked through and flakes easily when tested with a fork. Serve with the tomatoes.

Per Serving: Calories: 248; Protein: 23g; Cholesterol: 57mg; Sodium: 493mg; Total Carbohydrates: 3g; Fiber: 1g; Total Fat: 16g; Saturated Fat: 4g

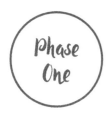

Phase One

PREP TIME: 10 MINUTES
COOK TIME: 15 MINUTES

1 medium head bok choy, leaves and stalks, thinly sliced and separated

1 red bell pepper, seeded and cut into strips

4 (4-ounce) cod fillets

1 (2-inch) piece fresh ginger, peeled and cut into matchsticks

2 scallions, white and green parts, thinly sliced

4 teaspoons tamari

4 teaspoons toasted sesame oil

Asian-Style Cod and Vegetables in Parchment

DAIRY-FREE | GRAIN-FREE | NUT-FREE | UNDER 30 MINUTES

Parchment paper is extremely useful in the kitchen. In these fish packets, it works as both the pan and the serving dish, minimizing your cleanup and locking in flavor. Served on a bed of bok choy and peppers, this is a filling dish. If you prefer, try it with different vegetables to create your own personalized packages. **SERVES 4**

1. Preheat the oven to 400°F.

2. Cut four large pieces of parchment paper and lay them on a large work surface.

3. On one side of each piece of parchment, place two large handfuls of bok choy (one handful of greens and one of stalks). On top of each, place several strips of bell pepper. Lay one cod fillet on each bed of vegetables. Place equal amounts of ginger sticks on the fish, arranging them evenly. Sprinkle with the scallions.

4. In a small bowl, whisk the tamari and sesame oil. Spoon 2 teaspoons of the sauce over each fillet.

5. Working with one piece of parchment, fold it over the top of the fish, fold the edges over, and crease to seal. Continue to work around the paper, closing the edges until you have a sealed package. Repeat with the remaining three pieces of parchment.

6. Arrange the packages on a large baking sheet and bake for 15 minutes. Remove from the oven and let the packages rest for a couple of minutes. Cut through the parchment to serve.

MAKE AHEAD These packets can be entirely assembled the night before and stored on a baking sheet in the refrigerator until you are ready to cook the following day.

Per Serving: Calories: 189; Protein: 27g; Cholesterol: 47mg; Sodium: 517mg; Total Carbohydrates: 4g; Fiber: 6g; Total Fat: 6g; Saturated Fat: 1g

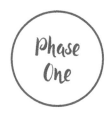

Phase One

PREP TIME: 10 MINUTES
COOK TIME: 15 MINUTES

10 ounces cremini
mushrooms, sliced

8 to 10 scallions, white
and green parts, cut into
2-inch segments

1 pound salmon fillets,
cut into 4 pieces

2 tablespoons extra-virgin
olive oil

1 tablespoon red or white
miso paste

1 tablespoon sake or other
dry cooking wine

Miso Salmon and Vegetables in Parchment

DAIRY-FREE | NUT-FREE | UNDER 30 MINUTES

In Japanese cuisine, miso is often combined with fish to impart a salty umami flavor. In this fish packet, it is combined with salmon, mushrooms, and scallions for an omega-3 burst of fatty acids. Serve the packages with Cauliflower Rice (page 188) or ½ cup of brown rice (see page 81). SERVES 4

1. Preheat the oven to 400°F.

2. Cut four large pieces of parchment paper and arrange on a large work surface.

3. Arrange one-fourth of the mushrooms on one side of each piece of parchment. Add equal amounts of scallions to each piece. Top each with a salmon fillet.

4. In a small bowl, whisk together the olive oil, miso paste, and sake. Pour an equal amount of sauce over each piece of fish.

5. Working with one piece of parchment, fold it over the top of the fish, fold the edges over, and crease to seal. Continue to work around the paper, closing the edges until you have a sealed package. Repeat with the remaining three pieces of parchment.

6. Arrange the packages on a large baking sheet and cook for 15 minutes. Remove from the oven and let the packages rest for a couple of minutes. Cut through the parchment to serve.

MAKE AHEAD These packets can be entirely assembled the night before and stored on a baking sheet in the refrigerator until you are ready to cook the following day.

Per Serving: Calories: 261; Protein: 26g; Cholesterol: 62mg; Sodium: 256mg; Total Carbohydrates: 6g; Fiber: 2g; Total Fat: 15g; Saturated Fat: 2g

Tilapia with Coconut Curry Sauce

DAIRY-FREE | GRAIN-FREE | NUT-FREE

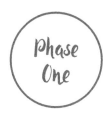

This Indian-style curry has coconut milk at its base and a warming blend of spices to raise it to the realm of luxurious. Loaded with healthy fat, this one-dish meal is quick to throw together. Serve this curry over Cauliflower Rice (page 188) or brown rice (see page 81). **SERVES 4**

PREP TIME: 10 MINUTES, PLUS 15 MINUTES TO MARINATE
COOK TIME: 15 MINUTES

2 tablespoons ground coriander, divided

¼ teaspoon ground turmeric

1 teaspoon cayenne pepper

1 pound tilapia fillets, cut into 1½-inch pieces

2 tablespoons coconut oil, divided

½ teaspoon mustard seeds

1 medium yellow onion, diced

½ teaspoon salt

1 green chile, stemmed and seeded

1 medium tomato, diced

1 cup light coconut milk

1. In a medium bowl, mix 1 tablespoon of coriander with the turmeric and cayenne pepper. Add the fish fillets and set them aside to marinate for 15 minutes.

2. In a large skillet, heat 1 tablespoon of coconut oil over medium-high heat and lightly fry the fish for about 3 minutes on each side. Remove the fish from skillet and set aside.

3. Add the remaining 1 tablespoon of coconut oil to the skillet and heat over medium-high heat. Add the mustard seeds and stir until they begin to pop, then add the onion and salt, and cook, stirring, for 2 minutes, until fragrant.

4. Add the remaining 1 tablespoon of coriander, the chile, and tomato and cook for 2 minutes, until the tomato begins to break down.

5. Add the coconut milk and 1 cup of water. Bring to a boil, then lower the heat and simmer for 5 minutes. Adjust the seasonings, adding a little more salt if needed. Return the fish to the curry and heat it through. Serve.

SUBSTITUTION TIP If you can't find tilapia, some great substitutions include red snapper, catfish, or flounder.

Per Serving: Calories: 244; Protein: 24g; Cholesterol: 57mg; Sodium: 354mg; Total Carbohydrates: 8g; Fiber: 2g; Total Fat: 14g; Saturated Fat: 10g

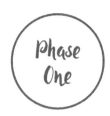

Phase One

PREP TIME: 15 MINUTES
COOK TIME: 10 MINUTES

2 tablespoons olive
   oil, divided
3 garlic cloves, minced
¼ teaspoon red
   pepper flakes
½ teaspoon salt, divided
1 pound large shrimp,
   shelled and deveined
¼ cup dry white wine
Juice of 1 lemon (about
   2 tablespoons), divided
2 tablespoons chopped
   fresh parsley
2 bunches kale, stemmed
   and coarsely chopped

Shrimp Scampi *and* Greens

DAIRY-FREE | GRAIN-FREE | NUT-FREE | UNDER 30 MINUTES

This classic shrimp dish can be given a healthier remake by dropping the processed noodles and serving the fragrant shrimp on a bed of kale instead. Seasoned with lemon, white wine, olive oil, and garlic, this delicious main course goes well with a side of Cauliflower Rice (page 188). **SERVES 4**

1. In a large skillet, heat 1 tablespoon of olive oil over medium-high heat. Add the garlic and red pepper flakes, and immediately reduce the heat to medium-low. Add ¼ teaspoon of salt to the skillet and mix well. Sauté the garlic for about 1 minute total, stirring constantly, until it just starts to brown.

2. Add the shrimp and wine, and stir to combine. Arrange the shrimp in a single layer. Increase the heat to high and bring to a boil for 2 minutes.

3. Flip the shrimp over and cook for 1 minute more.

4. Drizzle with 1 tablespoon of lemon juice and sprinkle with the parsley. Transfer to a serving dish to keep warm.

5. In the same skillet, heat the remaining 1 tablespoon of oil over medium-high heat. Add the kale and sauté for 3 to 5 minutes, stirring regularly, until it has wilted. Season with the remaining ¼ teaspoon of salt and 1 tablespoon of lemon juice. Serve the scampi over a bed of kale.

Per Serving: Calories: 202; Protein: 19g; Cholesterol: 142mg; Sodium: 980mg; Total Carbohydrates: 13g; Fiber: 4g; Total Fat: 9g; Saturated Fat: 1g

Blackened Cod *with* Pineapple Salsa

DAIRY-FREE | GRAIN-FREE | NUT-FREE | UNDER 30 MINUTES

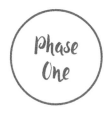

Phase One

Cod is a mild fish that pairs well with the bright fruit-forward flavors of this pineapple salsa. Using a blend of spices, the cod is blackened and smoky, providing a contrast to the cool, sweet salsa. **SERVES 4**

PREP TIME: 10 MINUTES
COOK TIME: 15 MINUTES

TO MAKE THE SALSA

In a small bowl, mix together the pineapple, bell pepper, tomato, cilantro, and scallions. Drizzle with the lime juice and the reserved pineapple juice and season with the salt and pepper.

TO MAKE THE FISH

1. Season the cod with the salt and pepper.

2. In a small bowl, mix together the paprika, onion powder, cayenne, thyme, and oregano. Use your hands to spread this mixture onto the fish.

3. In a large skillet, heat the oil over medium-high heat. Cook the fish on each side for 2 to 3 minutes, until it flakes easily when tested with a fork.

4. Serve topped with the pineapple salsa.

MAKE AHEAD Mix the salsa up to 1 day in advance and store in an airtight container in the refrigerator. Mix the seasoning mixture the night before, when making the salsa, for easy fish prep the next day.

Per Serving: Calories: 157; Protein: 21g; Cholesterol: 48mg; Sodium: 504mg; Total Carbohydrates: 10g; Fiber: 2g; Total Fat: 3g; Saturated Fat: 1g

FOR THE SALSA

1 (8-ounce) can pineapple in its own juices, drained, reserving 2 tablespoons juice

½ cup diced green bell pepper

1 small tomato, diced

¼ cup chopped fresh cilantro leaves

3 scallions, white and green parts, thinly sliced

Juice of 1 lime

¼ teaspoon salt

¼ teaspoon freshly ground black pepper

FOR THE FISH

1 pound cod fillets

½ teaspoon salt

Freshly ground black pepper

1 teaspoon smoked paprika

¼ teaspoon onion powder

¼ teaspoon cayenne pepper

¼ teaspoon dried thyme

¼ teaspoon dried oregano

2 teaspoons extra-virgin olive oil

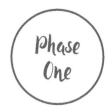

Phase One

PREP TIME: 10 MINUTES
COOK TIME: 6 MINUTES

1 pound tilapia fillets
Salt
Freshly ground
  black pepper
2 eggs
¾ cup almond flour
½ cup grated
  Parmesan cheese
1 teaspoon garlic powder
1 teaspoon extra-virgin
  olive oil
1 lemon, cut into wedges,
  for serving

Pan-Roasted Almond-Crusted Tilapia

GRAIN-FREE | UNDER 30 MINUTES

Almond flour provides a richness that other flours simply do not. While its high fat content can be prohibitive when baking and in other recipes where a large amount is needed, here the coating provides a match that is arguably even better than the flour or corn mixtures typically used to crust fish. SERVES 4

1. Season the tilapia with salt and pepper.

2. In a small bowl, beat the eggs.

3. In a separate small bowl, mix the almond flour, Parmesan, and garlic powder.

4. Dip each fillet into the egg, shake it to remove any excess egg, and press it into the flour mixture to cover.

5. In a skillet, heat the olive oil over medium-high heat. Add the fillets and cook for 3 minutes on one side, flip, and cook for 3 minutes more, until the fish flakes easily when tested with a fork. Serve with the lemon wedges.

Per Serving: Calories: 459; Protein: 40g; Cholesterol: 171mg; Sodium: 435mg; Total Carbohydrates: 10g; Fiber: 5g; Total Fat: 31g; Saturated Fat: 5g

One-Pan Salmon, Sweet Potato, and Brussels Sprouts Bake

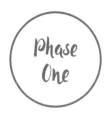

DAIRY-FREE | GRAIN-FREE | NUT-FREE | UNDER 30 MINUTES

PREP TIME: 10 MINUTES
COOK TIME: 20 MINUTES

For a boost of omega-3s, salmon is the best fish you can eat. Omega-3s are shown to reduce inflammation, lower the risk of chronic disease, and bolster brain and memory performance. This is an easy one-dish meal that leaves no mess. Simply toss everything on a baking sheet, pop it in the oven, and you are 20 minutes away from eating. Pour a glass of wine and relax! SERVES 4

1 pound salmon fillets

3 small sweet potatoes, roughly diced

1 pound Brussels sprouts, halved if large

2 teaspoons extra-virgin olive oil

1 teaspoon salt

½ teaspoon freshly ground black pepper

½ teaspoon garlic powder

¼ teaspoon dried thyme

1. Preheat the oven to 350°F.

2. Place the salmon in the middle of a large baking sheet. Arrange the sweet potatoes and Brussels sprouts around the salmon.

3. Drizzle the vegetables with the olive oil and use a spatula to stir them up a bit. Sprinkle the salt, pepper, garlic powder, and thyme over the fish and vegetables.

4. Bake for 20 minutes, until the fish flakes easily when tested with a fork and the vegetables are tender and lightly browned.

DID YOU KNOW? Parchment paper is simply paper that can withstand high cooking temperatures without burning. To make cleanup easier, line baking sheets with parchment paper and simply throw the mess away when you are done.

Per Serving: Calories: 317; Protein: 28g; Cholesterol: 62mg; Sodium: 714mg; Total Carbohydrates: 30g; Fiber: 7g; Total Fat: 10g; Saturated Fat: 2g

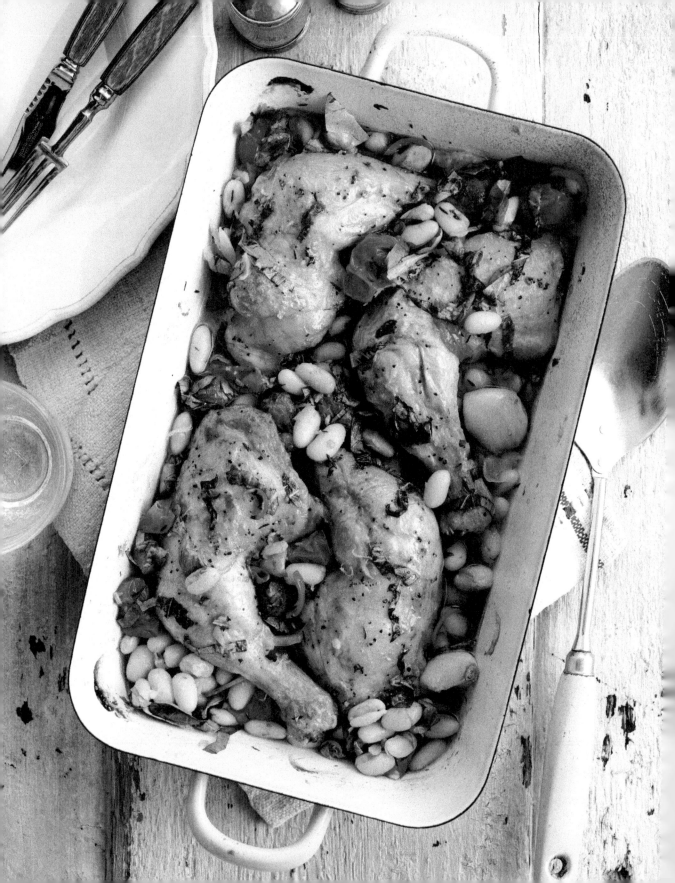

Meat and Poultry Mains

Once you are in phase two of the diet, meat is back on the table. However, it should not be in generous portions, but instead just an element of the meal. In the following recipes, you will find a variety of tempting ways to step away from large cuts like steaks and chops and instead serve up balanced, plant-strong courses with the savory flavors of meat to accent the meal.

« *Chicken, Tomatoes, and White Bean Bake (page 170)*

Simple Baked Chicken Breasts

DAIRY-FREE | GRAIN-FREE | NUT-FREE | UNDER 30 MINUTES

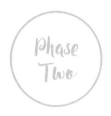

Phase Two

PREP TIME: 5 MINUTES
COOK TIME: 15 MINUTES

When you prepare chicken breasts in advance, it is easy to add some to meals to make a complete and nourishing main course in a matter of minutes. This simple recipe is designed for just this purpose. Make a batch, and you have chicken to use in four meals throughout the week. Adjust the recipe as needed for your weekly meal plan. **SERVES 8**

Nonstick cooking spray

2 pounds boneless skinless chicken breasts

1 teaspoon salt

1 teaspoon freshly ground black pepper

½ teaspoon garlic powder

½ teaspoon dried parsley

1. Preheat the oven to 400°F.

2. Spray a baking sheet with cooking spray.

3. Season the chicken with the salt, pepper, garlic, and parsley. Arrange the breasts on the baking sheet and bake for 35 minutes, until their juices run clear when pierced with a knife.

4. Let the chicken breasts cool completely and then transfer them to an airtight container. Refrigerate for up to 3 days or freeze for up to 1 month.

SUBSTITUTION TIP Use any of your favorite spices in this recipe to season the chicken to your liking. Cajun seasonings, lemon pepper, basil, thyme, and chili powder can all add great elements to chicken.

Per Serving: Calories: 102; Protein: 23g; Cholesterol: 61mg; Sodium: 524mg; Total Carbohydrates: 0g; Fiber: 0g; Total Fat: 2g; Saturated Fat: 0g

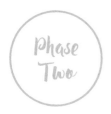

PREP TIME: 10 MINUTES

- 8 cups romaine, green or red leaf lettuce, or baby salad greens
- 8 ounces Simple Baked Chicken Breasts (page 159), cut into thin strips
- ½ cup crumbled feta cheese
- ¼ cup walnut pieces
- 2 clementines, peeled and segmented (see Tip)
- 2 celery stalks, thinly sliced on the diagonal
- 1 recipe Red Wine Vinaigrette (page 201), Bright Lemon-Garlic Vinaigrette (page 202), or Mustard Vinaigrette (page 203)

Easy Chicken Dinner Salad

GRAIN-FREE | UNDER 30 MINUTES

Making use of your precooked chicken breasts, this salad is super easy to throw together on a busy night. The combination of feta, walnuts, clementines, and celery provides a winning mix of sweet, salty, and crunchy, but the salad is easily customizable to whatever you like or have on hand. SERVES 4

1. On each of four plates, arrange 2 cups of lettuce. Divide the chicken, feta, walnuts, clementines, and celery slices equally between the four plates.

2. Top with 2 tablespoons of your preferred vinaigrette. Serve.

INGREDIENT TIP Clementines are a type of mandarin orange popular in the winter. Small and almost always seedless, clementines can be replaced with other mandarins such as satsumas. Tangerines also have a great flavor, but typically have many seeds, which would need to be removed.

Per Serving: Calories: 300; Protein: 16g; Cholesterol: 47mg; Sodium: 671mg; Total Carbohydrates: 9g; Fiber: 3g; Total Fat: 23g; Saturated Fat: 5g

Chicken *and* Quinoa Salad Bowl

UNDER 30 MINUTES

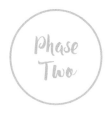

Phase Two

This is a warming salad bowl tied together with a generous serving of Yogurt Tahini Dressing to make a filling meal for lunch or dinner. Prep the quinoa in one big batch earlier in the week to have on hand to make this bowl come together in just a few minutes. **SERVES 4**

PREP TIME: 10 MINUTES

2 cups cooked quinoa

1 bunch kale, stemmed and cut into thin strips

1 tablespoon extra-virgin olive oil

8 ounces Simple Baked Chicken Breasts (page 159), cut into thin strips

1 recipe Yogurt Tahini Dressing (page 206)

2 tablespoons sesame seeds

1. In each of four bowls, put ½ cup quinoa.

2. In a mixing bowl, toss the kale and olive oil, massaging with your hands to work the oil into the leaves. Divide equally between the bowls. Divide the chicken equally between the bowls.

3. Top each bowl with 2 tablespoons of Yogurt Tahini Dressing and 1½ teaspoons of sesame seeds. Serve.

Per Serving: Calories: 348; Protein: 20g; Cholesterol: 33mg; Sodium: 406mg; Total Carbohydrates: 29g; Fiber: 5g; Total Fat: 19g; Saturated Fat: 3g

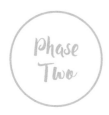

Phase Two

PREP TIME: 10 MINUTES

3 cups diced Simple
   Baked Chicken Breasts
   (page 159)

½ cup grapes, halved

1 celery stalk,
   finely chopped

2 tablespoons chopped
   fresh parsley

2 scallions, white and
   green parts, thinly sliced

⅓ cup unsweetened
   plain yogurt

2 tablespoons freshly
   squeezed lemon juice

¼ teaspoon salt

¼ teaspoon freshly ground
   black pepper

4 cups chopped romaine,
   red or green leaf lettuce,
   or baby salad greens

Chicken Salad
on a **Bed** *of* **Greens**

GRAIN-FREE | NUT-FREE | UNDER 30 MINUTES

Creamy chicken salad is a lunchtime comfort food classic. Here I use probiotic yogurt, along with grapes and celery, for a bit of crunchy sweetness. Served on a bed of lettuce, this is a filling meal that you can enjoy at any time of day. SERVES 4

1. In a bowl, toss together the chicken, grapes, celery, parsley, and scallions.

2. Add the yogurt, lemon juice, salt, and pepper. Stir to combine.

3. On each of four plates, place 1 cup of salad greens topped by 1 cup of chicken salad. Serve.

SUBSTITUTION TIP If you like a little zing, add a teaspoon or more of mustard or your favorite hot sauce to the salad in step 2.

Per Serving: Calories: 231; Protein: 27g; Cholesterol: 63mg; Sodium: 698mg; Total Carbohydrates: 8g; Fiber: 3g; Total Fat: 12g; Saturated Fat: 1g

Chinese Chicken Lettuce Wraps

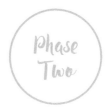

Phase Two

DAIRY-FREE | GRAIN-FREE | NUT-FREE | UNDER 30 MINUTES

PREP TIME: 10 MINUTES
COOK TIME: 5 MINUTES

Here is another easy quick-to-make recipe using cooked chicken. Served in lettuce wraps, this simple dish is perfectly paired with a side salad, or even some leftover roasted root vegetables for a heartier meal. **SERVES 4**

1 tablespoon extra-virgin olive oil

1 teaspoon sesame oil

2 tablespoons tamari

1 teaspoon honey

1 (1-inch) piece fresh ginger, minced

1 garlic clove, minced

2 cups Simple Baked Chicken Breasts, thinly sliced (page 159)

8 large lettuce leaves

1. In a medium saucepan over medium heat, combine the olive oil, sesame oil, tamari, honey, ginger, and garlic. Bring to a simmer and add the chicken, stirring to coat it in the sauce. Cook until just heated through, about 5 minutes.

2. Spoon ¼ cup of the cooked chicken into each lettuce leaf and serve.

Per Serving: Calories: 135; Protein: 19g; Cholesterol: 46mg; Sodium: 905mg; Total Carbohydrates: 3g; Fiber: 1g; Total Fat: 6g; Saturated Fat: 1g

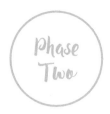

Phase Two

PREP TIME: 10 MINUTES
COOK TIME: 15 MINUTES

1 tomato, diced

2 tablespoons crumbled feta cheese

2 tablespoons pitted kalamata olives

1 tablespoon minced fresh basil leaves

4 boneless skinless chicken breasts

¼ teaspoon salt

¼ teaspoon freshly ground black pepper

1 tablespoon extra-virgin olive oil

Mediterranean Chicken Breasts

GRAIN-FREE | NUT-FREE | UNDER 30 MINUTES

The flavors of the Mediterranean come alive in this dish with feta, tomatoes, and kalamata olives. Stuffing chicken breasts is a great way to add flavor to a simple meal. **SERVES 4**

1. In a small bowl, combine the tomato, feta, olives, and basil.

2. Cut a horizontal slit in each chicken breast to create a pocket. Stuff about 2 tablespoons of the mixture into each chicken breast and close the opening with a wooden toothpick.

3. Season the chicken breasts with the salt and pepper.

4. In a large skillet, heat the olive oil over medium heat. Cook the chicken breasts for 12 to 15 minutes, flipping halfway through, until their juices run clear when pierced with a knife. Serve.

SUBSTITUTION TIP This recipe can be modified to fit your preferences. Basil and Parmesan create a good combination, as does a mix of tomatoes, scallions, cilantro, and freshly squeezed lime juice for a salsa-like stuffed breast.

Per Serving: Calories: 160; Protein: 24g; Cholesterol: 64mg; Sodium: 493mg; Total Carbohydrates: 2g; Fiber: 0g; Total Fat: 7g; Saturated Fat: 1g

Bok Choy *and* Chicken Stir-Fry

DAIRY-FREE | GRAIN-FREE | NUT-FREE

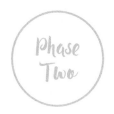

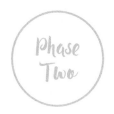

Phase
Two

Stir-fries are some of the easiest meals to make. Because everything is cooked together in one pan, dishes are minimized and you can focus on the main course. If you don't have a wok, use a flat-bottomed skillet instead. SERVES 4

PREP TIME: 10 MINUTES,
PLUS 20 MINUTES
TO MARINATE
COOK TIME: 10 MINUTES

2 tablespoons tamari

2 tablespoons rice vinegar

1 teaspoon sesame oil

1 teaspoon honey

1 (2-inch) piece fresh ginger, minced, divided

2 garlic cloves, minced, divided

½ pound boneless chicken thighs, thinly sliced

2 tablespoons canola oil, divided

1 large head bok choy, thinly sliced

1. In a medium bowl, combine the tamari, rice vinegar, sesame oil, and honey. Add half of the ginger and half of the garlic to the bowl, then add the chicken and turn it to coat.

2. In a wok, heat 1 tablespoon of canola oil over medium-high heat. Add the chicken (reserving the marinade) and cook, stirring constantly, for about 3 minutes, until cooked through. Transfer the chicken to a plate.

3. Add the remaining 1 tablespoon of oil to the wok and heat over medium-high heat. Add the bok choy and cook, stirring constantly, for 2 to 3 minutes, until it begins to soften and wilt.

4. Pour the marinade into the wok and stir with the bok choy to combine. Push the bok choy to the side of the wok and add the remaining ginger and garlic to the middle of the wok. Sauté briefly, until just fragrant, then mix it with the bok choy. Return the chicken to the wok and stir to combine. Serve.

Per Serving: Calories: 254; Protein: 22g; Cholesterol: 51mg; Sodium: 701mg; Total Carbohydrates: 5g; Fiber: 6g; Total Fat: 15g; Saturated Fat: 2g

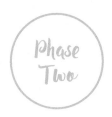

PREP TIME: 10 MINUTES
COOK TIME: 10 MINUTES

4 cups broccoli florets, cut to uniform size

8 ounces boneless skinless chicken breasts, thinly sliced

1 (2-inch) piece fresh ginger, minced, divided

2 tablespoons rice cooking wine or sake, divided

1 tablespoon tamari

½ teaspoon honey

2 tablespoons rice vinegar

2 tablespoons canola oil

4 garlic cloves, minced

1 red bell pepper, cut into thin strips

Chicken *and* Broccoli Stir-Fry

DAIRY-FREE | GRAIN-FREE | NUT-FREE | UNDER 30 MINUTES

This stir-fry is big on vegetables, combining broccoli and red pepper for a quick and delicious meal. Serve the stir-fry over Cauliflower Rice (page 188) or brown rice (see page 81). SERVES 4

1. Bring a large saucepan of water to a boil over high heat. Add the broccoli florets, and when the water returns to a boil, set a timer for 1 minute. Drain the broccoli in a colander, and leave it over the sink to drain further.

2. In a large bowl, combine the chicken, half of the ginger, 1 tablespoon of rice wine, the tamari, and the honey.

3. In a small bowl, combine ¼ cup of water, the remaining 1 tablespoon of rice wine, and the rice vinegar.

4. In a large wok or skillet, heat the canola oil over medium-high heat. Lift the chicken pieces out of the marinade, add them to the wok, and sear them for 1 minute undisturbed, before stirring and adding the garlic and remaining ginger. Continue to stir for about 1 minute, until the chicken has mostly changed color but is not completely cooked through.

5. Add the rice wine mixture along with the red pepper and broccoli to the wok. Stir-fry for 2 minutes, until the chicken is cooked through and the broccoli is fork-tender.

SUBSTITUTION TIP Vegetables can be substituted here as desired; just be sure to use fresh vegetables, or in some cases canned, for the most flavor and best texture in a wok. Snow peas, thinly sliced carrots, mushrooms, water chestnuts, and baby corn all work well in this dish.

Per Serving: Calories: 178; Protein: 15g; Cholesterol: 30mg; Sodium: 399mg; Total Carbohydrates: 12g; Fiber: 3g; Total Fat: 8g; Saturated Fat: 1g

Chicken and Root Vegetable Roast

DAIRY-FREE | GRAIN-FREE | NUT-FREE

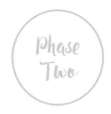

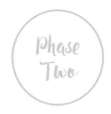Phase Two

Sometimes cooking a one-pan meal is all you have the energy for. If that's the case, this chicken and root vegetable roast is the answer. You can simply brown the chicken breasts for flavor, throw it all in a pan, and set the timer. Pour yourself a glass of wine and catch up on some reading while you wait. SERVES 4

PREP TIME: 10 MINUTES
COOK TIME: 35 MINUTES

1 pound small turnips, cut into 1-inch chunks
½ pound sweet potatoes, cut into 1-inch chunks
1 tablespoon fresh rosemary, chopped
2 tablespoons extra-virgin olive oil, divided
½ teaspoon salt, divided
½ teaspoon freshly ground black pepper, divided
2 bone-in chicken breasts, cut in half crosswise

1. Preheat the oven to 450°F.

2. In a large bowl, toss together the turnips, sweet potatoes, rosemary, 1 tablespoon of olive oil, ¼ teaspoon of salt, and ¼ teaspoon of pepper. Spread the mixture on a baking sheet in a single layer. Roast for 15 minutes.

3. While the vegetables are roasting, season the chicken with the remaining ¼ teaspoon salt and remaining ¼ teaspoon of pepper.

4. In a large skillet, heat the remaining 1 tablespoon of oil over medium-high heat. Place the chicken pieces skin-side down in the skillet and sear for about 5 minutes, until browned and crisp. Remove from the heat.

5. When the vegetables have roasted for 15 minutes, remove the baking sheet and stir the vegetables. Place the chicken pieces, skin-side up, on the baking sheet and return to the oven for 20 minutes more, until the vegetables are tender and the chicken is cooked through. Serve.

SUBSTITUTION TIP If you can't find whole chicken breasts, substitute whole thighs instead. Be sure to trim off any excess fat before cooking.

Per Serving: Calories: 308; Protein: 20g; Cholesterol: 56mg; Sodium: 453mg; Total Carbohydrates: 23g; Fiber: 4g; Total Fat: 15g; Saturated Fat: 3g

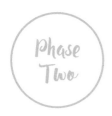

PREP TIME: 10 MINUTES,
PLUS OVERNIGHT
TO MARINATE
COOK TIME: 40 MINUTES

⅓ cup freshly squeezed
   lemon juice

1 tablespoon honey

2 teaspoons
   ground cinnamon

½ teaspoon red
   pepper flakes

1 teaspoon salt

½ teaspoon freshly ground
   black pepper

2 teaspoons ground cumin

1 teaspoon smoked paprika

½ cup pitted green
   kalamata olives

¼ cup dried apricots, diced

½ cup chopped
   fresh cilantro

1 pound chicken legs
   (thighs and/or drumsticks)

Chicken, Apricot, and Olive Bake

DAIRY-FREE | GRAIN-FREE | NUT-FREE

Sweet and salty flavors combine in this lemon-infused one-pan bake. Prep this the night before to let it marinate overnight, and the following day all you will have to do is pour it into the pan and look forward to dinner. **SERVES 4**

1. In a large bowl, whisk the lemon juice, honey, cinnamon, red pepper flakes, salt, pepper, cumin, and paprika together. Add the olives, apricots, cilantro, and chicken. Mix well. Transfer to a zippered plastic bag or airtight container and refrigerate overnight, up to 24 hours.

2. Preheat the oven to 375°F.

3. Transfer the chicken and all the marinade ingredients to a baking dish. Bake for 40 minutes, until the chicken juices run clear when pierced with a knife. Serve.

Per Serving: Calories: 362; Protein: 30g; Cholesterol: 104mg; Sodium: 650mg; Total Carbohydrates: 15g; Fiber: 2g; Total Fat: 20g; Saturated Fat: 4g

Cauliflower Rice Chicken Biriyani

DAIRY-FREE | GRAIN-FREE | UNDER 30 MINUTES

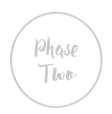

Phase Two

Biriyani is a South Asian rice dish that combines rice, vegetables or meat, and spices. The delectable collision of flavors is memorable, and in this reworked version using cauliflower rice, it holds up well to the original. **SERVES 4**

PREP TIME: 10 MINUTES
COOK TIME: 15 MINUTES

1. In a large skillet, heat the olive oil over medium-high heat and cook the onion for 3 to 5 minutes, until it begins to soften.

2. Add the chicken, carrot, garlic, ginger, cumin, turmeric, and cinnamon and stir constantly for 1 to 2 minutes, until the chicken is browned on the outside and the spices are fragrant but not burnt.

3. Add the chicken stock, cauliflower, and salt. Stir to combine and bring to a simmer.

4. Reduce the heat to medium, cover the skillet, and cook for 10 minutes, until the chicken is cooked through. If there is still some broth in the pan, remove the lid and let it cook down so that the "rice" is dry. Serve, topped with the cashews and cilantro.

MAKE AHEAD Biriyani actually tastes better when the flavors are able to meld together. Make this up to 2 days in advance and store it in an airtight container in the refrigerator. When you want to serve it, reheat it in a saucepan on the stove or in a microwave-safe dish in the microwave.

Per Serving: Calories: 244; Protein: 20g; Cholesterol: 30mg; Sodium: 502mg; Total Carbohydrates: 21g; Fiber: 6g; Total Fat: 11g; Saturated Fat: 2g

1 tablespoon extra-virgin olive oil

1 large yellow onion, finely chopped

2 boneless skinless chicken breasts, diced

1 carrot, finely chopped

2 garlic cloves, minced

1 (1-inch) piece fresh ginger, minced

1 teaspoon ground cumin

1 teaspoon ground turmeric

½ teaspoon ground cinnamon

1 cup low-sodium chicken stock

1 large head cauliflower, shredded on a box grater or in a food processor

½ teaspoon salt

¼ cup cashews, for serving

½ cup chopped fresh cilantro leaves, for serving

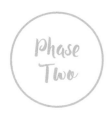

PREP TIME: 10 MINUTES
COOK TIME: 1 HOUR

2 bone-in chicken quarters

½ teaspoon salt, divided

½ teaspoon freshly ground
black pepper, divided

1 tablespoon canola oil

1 red bell pepper,
coarsely chopped

4 shallots, halved

2 garlic cloves

1 rosemary sprig, stem
removed and leaves
roughly chopped

1 cup low-sodium
chicken stock

1 cup chopped chard leaves

2 (15-ounce) cans
butter beans

Chicken, Tomatoes, and White Bean Bake

DAIRY-FREE | GRAIN-FREE | NUT-FREE

If you want your house to smell great, this is a wonderful recipe to try. There is nothing quite like the smell of chicken baking, and when rosemary is in the equation, it is all the better. The combination of chicken and beans provides a high-fiber, protein-packed meal that is a terrific way to end your day. SERVES 4

1. Preheat the oven to 375°F.

2. Season the chicken with ¼ teaspoon of salt and ¼ teaspoon of pepper.

3. In a large saucepan, heat the canola oil over medium-high heat and brown the chicken pieces on both sides. Remove them from the saucepan and set them aside.

4. Add the bell pepper, shallots, garlic, and rosemary to the saucepan and cook for 3 minutes, stirring regularly. Add the stock and chard, reduce the heat to medium, and bring to a simmer for 5 minutes. Add the beans, the remaining ¼ teaspoon of salt, and the remaining ¼ teaspoon of pepper.

5. Transfer the bean mixture to a large baking dish. Top with the chicken quarters.

6. Bake for 40 to 45 minutes, until the chicken is cooked through and its juices run clear when pierced with a knife. Serve.

Per Serving: Calories: 426; Protein: 34g; Cholesterol: 119mg; Sodium: 478mg; Total Carbohydrates: 22g; Fiber: 5g; Total Fat: 22g; Saturated Fat: 5g

Herb-Crusted Chicken Thighs *and* Polenta

DAIRY-FREE

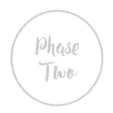

Chicken thighs are fatty, but that doesn't mean you need to avoid them altogether. Instead, work to make them the best they can be by removing the skin and trimming the fat. This recipe uses a lemon-herb crust to add flavor, and the chicken is served on a bed of creamy polenta for a filling meal that you can feel good about. **SERVES 4**

PREP TIME: 10 MINUTES
COOK TIME: 25 MINUTES

FOR THE CHICKEN
Nonstick cooking spray
Juice of 2 lemons
1 tablespoon freshly grated
  lemon zest
4 garlic cloves, minced
½ teaspoon dried rosemary
½ teaspoon dried thyme
¼ teaspoon salt
1 tablespoon extra-virgin
  olive oil
1 pound bone-in chicken
  thighs, skin removed

FOR THE POLENTA
2 cups unsweetened plain
  almond milk
½ cup uncooked
  quick-cooking polenta
  (see Tip)
¼ teaspoon salt

TO MAKE THE CHICKEN
1. Preheat the oven to 350°F.

2. Spray a baking dish with nonstick cooking spray.

3. In a bowl, combine the lemon juice, lemon zest, garlic, rosemary, thyme, salt, and olive oil. Add the chicken thighs and turn them to coat well. Transfer the thighs and liquid to the baking dish, spooning the herbs and garlic on top of the thighs.

4. Cover with aluminum foil and bake for 20 to 25 minutes, until the chicken is cooked through and its juices run clear when pierced with a knife.

TO MAKE THE POLENTA
In a small saucepan over medium heat, bring the almond milk and ⅓ cup of water to a simmer. Add the polenta in a slow stream, whisking constantly. Continue stirring for 3 minutes, until the polenta has thickened. Stir in the salt. Serve the polenta topped with the chicken thighs.

INGREDIENT TIP Polenta is a dish made from coarsely ground corn-meal. Select a quick-cooking variety to have the dish complete in a matter of minutes. Traditional polenta requires about 40 minutes of constant stirring, making the quick-cook variety, which takes only a few minutes, a great time-saver.

Per Serving: Calories: 350; Protein: 31g; Cholesterol: 107mg; Sodium: 486mg; Total Carbohydrates: 15g; Fiber: 2g; Total Fat: 18g; Saturated Fat: 4g

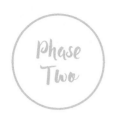

PREP TIME: 10 MINUTES
COOK TIME: 40 MINUTES

½ large head cauliflower, broken into small florets (4 to 6 cups)

8 ounces lean ground beef

2 tablespoons extra-virgin olive oil

1 yellow onion, diced

2 green bell peppers, diced

1 (15-ounce) can whole tomatoes

½ teaspoon salt

¼ teaspoon freshly ground black pepper

1 tablespoon tomato paste

½ cup shredded mozzarella cheese

Beef *and* Cauliflower Bake

GRAIN-FREE | NUT-FREE

This is a comfort food casserole that just goes to show you delicious food can still be good for you. Loaded with cauliflower, this baked entrée has the meaty greatness of the casseroles of your childhood, but with about half the actual meat. Instead, vegetables bulk up the bake and you won't miss a thing. SERVES 4

1. Preheat the oven to 350°F.

2. Fill a large saucepan with a couple of inches of water. Place a steamer basket in the saucepan and bring the water to a boil over high heat. Add the cauliflower to the steamer basket (making sure the water does not touch the vegetables) and cook for 8 to 10 minutes, until fork-tender.

3. In a skillet over medium heat, cook the beef until thoroughly browned. Drain and discard any oil from the meat.

4. Add the olive oil, onion, and bell peppers to the skillet and cook, stirring regularly, for 3 minutes. Add the tomatoes, breaking them apart with the spoon as you stir them in. Season with the salt and pepper, and continue to cook for 3 minutes more.

5. In a small bowl, combine the tomato paste with ½ cup of water and stir. Pour this into the skillet and cook for 5 minutes more.

6. In a baking dish, arrange the cauliflower on the bottom. Sprinkle half of the mozzarella on the cauliflower. Top with the beef mixture and then the remaining cheese. Bake for 20 minutes. Let the casserole rest for 5 minutes before serving.

MAKE AHEAD Make and assemble the casserole through to topping it with cheese, then cover and let it cool to room temperature. Refrigerate it overnight and bake it the following day, adding about 5 minutes to the cooking time to account for it coming out of the refrigerator.

Per Serving: Calories: 366; Protein: 26g; Cholesterol: 68mg; Sodium: 683mg; Total Carbohydrates: 15g; Fiber: 5g; Total Fat: 23g; Saturated Fat: 8g

Mushroom Beef Burger Lettuce Wrap

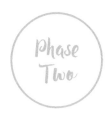

DAIRY-FREE | GRAIN-FREE | NUT-FREE | UNDER 30 MINUTES

Mushrooms have a texture and color similar to beef, allowing them to mingle well while significantly cutting back the calories and fat in the dish. These delicious burgers are easy to whip up and have on the table in under 30 minutes, making them perfect for a weeknight meal. Serve them wrapped in lettuce for a microbiome-friendly main dish that satisfies. **SERVES 4**

PREP TIME: 5 MINUTES
COOK TIME: 15 MINUTES

10 ounces cremini mushrooms

1 tablespoon extra-virgin olive oil

¼ cup finely diced yellow onion

½ teaspoon salt

½ teaspoon freshly ground black pepper

8 ounces lean ground beef

1 egg, beaten

4 large lettuce leaves, for serving

4 tomato slices, for serving

Ketchup (page 199), or store-bought, for serving

Mustard, for serving

1. In a food processor, pulse the mushrooms until coarsely ground.

2. In a large skillet, heat the olive oil over medium-high heat and sauté the mushrooms, onion, salt, and pepper for about 5 minutes, until the vegetables begin to brown and soften. Transfer them to a bowl to cool.

3. When the mushroom mixture is cool, add the beef and egg. Mix together well and form into four patties.

4. Wipe the skillet clean with a paper towel and heat over medium heat. Add the burgers and fry for 4 to 5 minutes per side, until cooked through.

5. Place each burger on a lettuce leaf, top each with a tomato slice and some Ketchup and mustard, and wrap the leaf around the burger to serve.

Per Serving: Calories: 241; Protein: 13g; Cholesterol: 94mg; Sodium: 356mg; Total Carbohydrates: 4g; Fiber: 1g; Total Fat: 19g; Saturated Fat: 6g

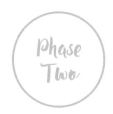

PREP TIME: 5 MINUTES
COOK TIME: 6 TO 8 HOURS
ON LOW

FOR THE BEEF

1 small yellow onion, diced

2 pounds flank steak

2 tablespoons honey

¼ cup tamari

1 (2-inch) piece fresh
ginger, grated

2 tablespoons rice vinegar

1 teaspoon sesame oil

FOR THE SLAW

2 cups red cabbage,
shredded

1 tablespoon tamari

2 tablespoons rice vinegar

FOR SERVING

16 lettuce leaves

Slow Cooker Korean Beef Tacos with Red Slaw

DAIRY-FREE | GRAIN-FREE | NUT-FREE

The great thing about a slow cooker meal is that it is ready when you are. Throw these ingredients in the slow cooker in the morning, and you will come home to an awesome aroma and have dinner mostly complete. Whip up the three-ingredient slaw, and dinner is served. SERVES 8

TO MAKE THE BEEF

1. Lay the onion on the bottom of the slow cooker. Top with the flank steak.

2. In a small bowl, mix the honey, tamari, ginger, rice vinegar, and sesame oil. Pour the mixture over the meat. Flip the steak once or twice to coat.

3. Cover and cook on low for 6 to 8 hours (or on high for 4 to 6 hours), until you are able to easily shred the meat with two forks.

4. Shred the meat.

TO MAKE THE SLAW

In a bowl, combine the cabbage, tamari, and rice vinegar. Toss well.

TO SERVE

Fill the lettuce leaves with 2 tablespoons of meat, topped by 2 tablespoons of slaw. Serve.

MAKE AHEAD The meat mixture can be made up to 2 days ahead and reheated in a saucepan on the stove or in the microwave. Do not assemble the tacos until ready to serve to prevent them from becoming soggy.

Per Serving: Calories: 200; Protein: 26g; Cholesterol: 70mg; Sodium: 700mg; Total Carbohydrates: 8g; Fiber: 1g; Total Fat: 7g; Saturated Fat: 2g

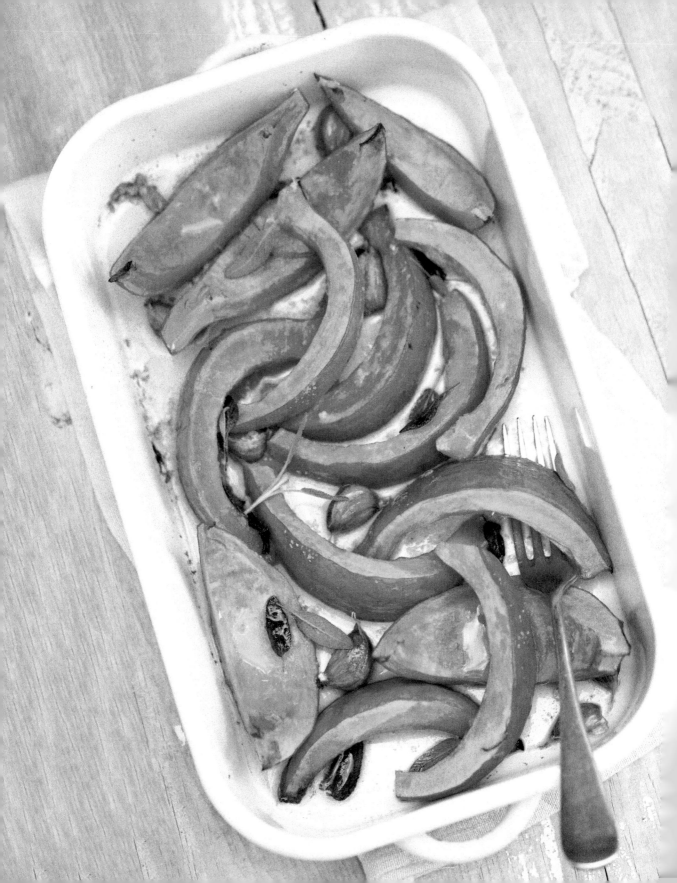

Snacks and Sides

This chapter is dedicated to the smaller bites that accompany dishes or tide you over between meals. Featuring a wide variety of simple veggie-forward snacks and sides, this chapter gives you plenty of ideas that are easy to whip up while dinner is cooking. Pair them with mains to build healthy and well-balanced meals, or keep them on hand for curbing hunger.

Eggplant Yogurt Dip
with Vegetables

GRAIN-FREE | NUT-FREE

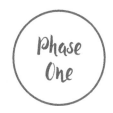

Eggplant is high in fiber, making it a great vegetable to add to your diet. You may find different varieties of eggplant at the grocery store, including thinner Asian varieties. For this recipe, use the larger version, which has a greater flesh-to-skin ratio. SERVES 8

1. Preheat the broiler.

2. Using a fork, poke several holes in the eggplant and place it on a baking sheet. Broil the eggplant for a total of 20 to 30 minutes, flipping it every 5 to 6 minutes, until the skin is charred in spots and the eggplant begins to deflate. Remove from the oven and let it cool.

3. Cut the eggplant in half lengthwise and use a spoon to scoop out the flesh. Transfer to a cutting board and finely chop the flesh. Discard the skin.

4. In a bowl, add the eggplant, yogurt, garlic, salt, and mint leaves. Stir to combine.

5. Serve with the bell peppers, cauliflower, and cucumbers for dipping.

Per Serving: Calories: 121; Protein: 7g; Cholesterol: 18mg; Sodium: 234mg; Total Carbohydrates: 16g; Fiber: 3g; Total Fat: 4g; Saturated Fat: 3g

PREP TIME: 10 MINUTES
COOK TIME: 30 MINUTES

1 large globe eggplant

1 quart low-fat plain yogurt

1 garlic clove, minced

½ teaspoon salt

2 or 3 fresh mint leaves, finely chopped

1 red bell pepper, cut into strips, for serving

1 green bell pepper, cut into strips, for serving

1 small head cauliflower, broken into florets, for serving

2 cucumbers, seeded and cut into spears, for serving

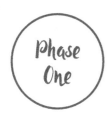

Phase One

PREP TIME: 10 MINUTES
COOK TIME: 45 MINUTES

2 medium beets, washed
  and trimmed (see Tip)
2 tablespoons extra-virgin
  olive oil, divided
½ cup unsweetened
  plain yogurt
2 tablespoons freshly
  squeezed lemon juice
1 garlic clove
1 teaspoon salt
½ teaspoon ground cumin

Beet Dip

GRAIN-FREE | NUT-FREE

This smooth red dip is great paired with crisp vegetables, such as radishes, carrots, jicama, and kohlrabi. Yogurt gives it a luxurious creamy texture and packs it full of healthy microbes for your gut. **MAKES 2 CUPS**

1. Preheat the oven to 350°F.

2. Place the beets on a large sheet of aluminum foil. Drizzle the beets with 2 teaspoons of olive oil and wrap them in the foil.

3. Bake for 45 minutes, until tender when pierced with a fork. When cool enough to handle, peel the beets.

4. In a blender, combine the beets, the remaining 4 teaspoons of olive oil, the yogurt, lemon juice, garlic, salt, and cumin. Serve.

INGREDIENT TIP Beets should be firm and plump when you buy them. If you purchase them together with their greens, you should remove the greens at their base when you get home and store them separately. Use beet greens as a substitution for chard in recipes.

Per Serving (¼ cup): Calories: 59; Protein: 1g; Cholesterol: 2mg; Sodium: 332mg; Total Carbohydrates: 5g; Fiber: 1g; Total Fat: 4g; Saturated Fat: 1g

Asparagus Hummus

DAIRY-FREE | GRAIN-FREE | NUT-FREE | VEGAN | UNDER 30 MINUTES

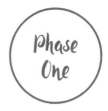

Phase One

PREP TIME: 10 MINUTES
COOK TIME: 5 MINUTES

This bright and sunny dip goes extremely well with fresh vegetables such as carrots, celery, cucumbers, and tomatoes. It also works nicely with the Almond Flour Crackers (page 184) for a complementary crunch to fight midday hunger. **MAKES 2 CUPS**

½ pound asparagus, trimmed and cut into 1-inch pieces

1 (15-ounce) can chickpeas, drained and rinsed

3 garlic cloves

2 tablespoons freshly squeezed lemon juice

2 tablespoons tahini (see Tip)

½ teaspoon salt

2 tablespoons extra-virgin olive oil

1. Bring a large saucepan of water to a boil over high heat. Fill a large mixing bowl with ice water.

2. Add the asparagus to the boiling water and cook for 3 minutes. Drain in a colander and transfer the asparagus to the ice bath.

3. In a blender, combine the chickpeas, garlic, lemon juice, tahini, and salt. Process until smooth. Add the cooled asparagus and process again until smooth. With the blender running, drizzle in the oil in a slow stream until mixed. Serve, or store in an airtight container in the refrigerator for up to 3 days.

INGREDIENT TIP Tahini is ground sesame paste. It can be found near the other nut and seed butters at the grocery store, or you can make it yourself by processing sesame seeds in a high-powdered blender until creamy.

Per Serving (¼ cup): Calories: 102; Protein: 4g; Cholesterol: 0mg; Sodium: 218mg; Total Carbohydrates: 9g; Fiber: 3g; Total Fat: 6g; Saturated Fat: 1g

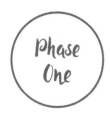

PREP TIME: 10 MINUTES
COOK TIME: 15 MINUTES

2 red peppers, halved, stemmed, and seeded (see Tip)
1 (15-ounce) can chickpeas, drained and rinsed
1 garlic clove
¼ cup freshly squeezed lemon juice
2 tablespoons extra-virgin olive oil
2 tablespoons tahini
½ teaspoon salt

Roasted Red Pepper Hummus

DAIRY-FREE | GRAIN-FREE | NUT-FREE | VEGAN | UNDER 30 MINUTES

Red peppers add more than just a dash of bright color to this quick hummus recipe. Their flavor, brought out through roasting, makes the hummus pop with character. Charring the peppers well before you remove them from the broiler will help you peel the skins off easily. **MAKES 2 CUPS**

1. Preheat the broiler.

2. Arrange the red peppers, skin-side up, on a baking sheet. Broil for 10 minutes, until the skin is blackened and charred. Remove from the oven and transfer to a covered container to steam for 3 to 5 minutes.

3. Use your fingers to remove the skin from the peppers. It should easily peel off. Transfer the peppers to a blender.

4. Add the chickpeas, garlic, lemon juice, olive oil, tahini, and salt. Process until smooth. Serve.

SUBSTITUTION TIP If you want to save a few minutes, use about ¾ cup of canned roasted red peppers.

Per Serving (¼ cup): Calories: 111; Protein: 3g; Cholesterol: 0mg; Sodium: 219mg; Total Carbohydrates: 11g; Fiber: 3g; Total Fat: 6g; Saturated Fat: 1g

Cinnamon Almonds

DAIRY-FREE | GRAIN-FREE

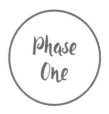

Phase One

This easy, make-ahead recipe elevates almonds to new heights. Egg whites help the spices stick to the almonds, and toasting the nuts and cinnamon deepens their flavors. **MAKES 2 CUPS**

PREP TIME: 5 MINUTES
COOK TIME: 1 HOUR

1 egg white
2 tablespoons ground cinnamon
Pinch salt
2 cups whole almonds

1. Preheat the oven to 250°F.

2. Line a baking sheet with parchment paper.

3. In a medium bowl, whisk the egg white until frothy. Add the cinnamon and salt and mix well.

4. Add the almonds and stir to coat. Transfer to the prepared baking sheet and shake the tray so the nuts settle in a single layer.

5. Bake for 1 hour, stirring every 15 minutes.

6. Cool the nuts completely, then transfer them to an airtight container for storage. Store at room temperature for 1 week.

SUBSTITUTION TIP Use any of your favorite spices to create your own spiced almonds. Nutmeg, clove, and allspice all offer warming touches, while curry powder, garlic powder, and onion powder can create savory nut combinations.

Per Serving (2 tablespoons): Calories: 106; Protein: 4g; Cholesterol: 0mg; Sodium: 13mg; Total Carbohydrates: 5g; Fiber: 3g; Total Fat: 9g; Saturated Fat: 1g

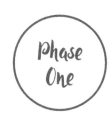

PREP TIME: 15 MINUTES
COOK TIME: 10 MINUTES

FOR THE CRACKERS

½ cup almond flour

½ cup flaxseed meal

¼ teaspoon salt

1½ teaspoons extra-virgin
olive oil

1 egg, beaten

**FOR THE HERBED
GOAT CHEESE**

2 ounces soft goat cheese

1 teaspoon minced
fresh rosemary

1 teaspoon minced
fresh thyme

Almond Flour Crackers *with* Herbed Goat Cheese

GRAIN-FREE | UNDER 30 MINUTES

Almond flour makes for a tasty, crunchy, high-fiber, gluten-free cracker. Bolstered with flaxseed meal, these crackers are loaded with omega-3s and make a wonderful snack when slathered with the herbed goat cheese. SERVES 4

TO MAKE THE CRACKERS

1. Preheat the oven to 400°F.

2. In a medium bowl, combine the almond flour, flaxseed meal, and salt. Toss well. Drizzle the olive oil over the mixture and add the egg. Stir to form a dough. If necessary, add 1 to 2 tablespoons of water.

3. Form the dough into a disc and place between two sheets of parchment paper. Using a rolling pin, roll the disc to about ¼-inch thickness. Remove the top layer of parchment and flip the dough over onto a large baking sheet. Remove the second layer of parchment. Using a pizza cutter, cut the dough into individual crackers. (This should yield about 25 non-uniform pieces, depending on how the dough is cut.)

4. Bake for 10 to 12 minutes, until crisp, keeping a watchful eye for darkening. Remove from the oven and let them cool on a wire rack. Store at room temperature in a covered container for up to 3 days.

TO MAKE THE HERBED GOAT CHEESE

In a small bowl, mix together the goat cheese, rosemary, and thyme. Store in an airtight container in the refrigerator for up to 3 days.

Per Serving: Calories: 380; Protein: 15g; Cholesterol: 59mg; Sodium: 226mg; Total Carbohydrates: 13g; Fiber: 9g; Total Fat: 33g; Saturated Fat: 5g

Sunchoke Chips

DAIRY-FREE | GRAIN-FREE | NUT-FREE | VEGAN

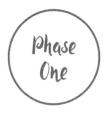

Unlike most root vegetables, sunchokes, or Jerusalem artichokes as they are also known, do not contain starchy carbohydrates. Instead, they are high in inulin, a prebiotic food that is beneficial for the microbiome and does not make blood sugar spike. With a mild, nutty flavor, these chips are perfect as an accompaniment to lunch or a quick snack during a long afternoon. If you don't have a mandolin, use a knife and take the time to make the slices as uniform as possible to promote even browning. SERVES 4

PREP TIME: 10 MINUTES
COOK TIME: 25 MINUTES

1 pound sunchokes, peeled
1 tablespoon coconut
   oil, melted
½ teaspoon salt

1. Preheat the oven to 400°F.

2. Line a baking sheet with parchment paper.

3. Wash the sunchokes well, removing any dirt with a kitchen brush. Using a mandolin, slice them into ¼-inch-thick rounds.

4. In a large bowl, toss the sunchoke rounds with the coconut oil. Sprinkle with the salt and toss again to combine.

5. Arrange the sunchokes on the baking sheet in a single layer. Bake for 15 minutes, then flip them and bake for an additional 10 minutes, keeping a watchful eye on the chips until they are browned and crisp. Serve within 3 to 4 hours of making.

Per Serving: Calories: 103; Protein: 2g; Cholesterol: 0mg; Sodium: 296mg;
Total Carbohydrates: 13g; Fiber: 4g; Total Fat: 4g; Saturated Fat: 3g

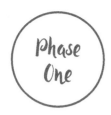

Phase One

PREP TIME: 10 MINUTES
COOK TIME: 30 MINUTES

2 large sweet potatoes
1 tablespoon coconut
   oil, melted
½ teaspoon salt

Sweet Potato Chips

DAIRY-FREE | GRAIN-FREE | NUT-FREE | VEGAN

Sweet potatoes, with their bright orange flesh, pack in carotenoid antioxidants and help stabilize blood sugar levels and the body's response to insulin. For these reasons, snacking on them makes more sense than the traditional white potato chip. Because they are also higher in natural sugars than white potatoes, they can satisfy a sweet tooth as well. SERVES 4

1. Preheat the oven to 375°F.

2. Line a baking sheet with parchment paper.

3. Using a mandolin or a sharp knife, slice the sweet potatoes into ¼-inch-thick rounds.

4. In a large bowl, toss the rounds with the coconut oil. Sprinkle with the salt and toss again to combine.

5. Arrange the sweet potato rounds on the baking sheet in a single layer. Bake for 10 minutes, then flip them. Bake for an additional 10 minutes. Then continue to cook the sweet potatoes for a final 10 minutes, this time checking them every minute or so for browning. Once browned, remove the chips from the oven and serve within 3 to 4 hours of making.

SUBSTITUTION TIP For even more flavor, add any of your favorite dried seasonings or herbs to these chips. Garlic powder offers a nice contrast, while thyme, rosemary, and sage pair well with the flavor of sweet potatoes.

Per Serving: Calories: 85; Protein: 1g; Cholesterol: 0mg; Sodium: 326mg; Total Carbohydrates: 13g; Fiber: 2g; Total Fat: 3g; Saturated Fat: 3g

Fruit *and* Nut Trail Mix

DAIRY-FREE | GRAIN-FREE | VEGAN | UNDER 30 MINUTES

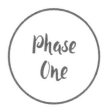

Phase One

The nuts and seeds in this trail mix are a good source of fat and protein, and the inclusion of dried fruit can satisfy your sweet tooth. Make a batch and enjoy it throughout the week as an easy snack when you need one. **SERVES 4**

PREP TIME: 5 MINUTES
COOK TIME: 10 MINUTES

½ cup raw almonds

¼ cup raw walnut halves

¼ cup raw sunflower seeds

¼ cup golden raisins

¼ cup dried
  apricots, halved

1. Preheat the oven to 350°F.

2. Spread the almonds, walnuts, and sunflower seeds on a baking sheet and toast for 10 minutes, shaking the tray once halfway through. Let the nuts cool completely on the baking sheet.

3. In a bowl, toss the nuts with the raisins and apricots. Store for up to 5 days in an airtight container at room temperature.

SUBSTITUTION TIP Mix and match any of your favorite dried fruits; just avoid those that are sweetened. Dried apples, cherries, goji berries, blueberries, strawberries, banana chips, figs, and dates all make great additions to trail mix. Be sure to keep the same proportions of 1 cup of nuts to ½ cup of fruit.

SUBSTITUTION TIP Pistachios, cashews, and peanuts are also great alternatives for the nuts. Whichever you buy, choose those that are raw, unsalted, unsweetened, and free of added oil.

Per Serving: Calories: 285; Protein: 8g; Cholesterol: 0mg; Sodium: 4mg; Total Carbohydrates: 29g; Fiber: 5g; Total Fat: 18g; Saturated Fat: 2g

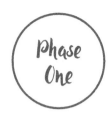

Phase One

PREP TIME: 10 MINUTES
COOK TIME: 10 MINUTES

1 large head cauliflower
1½ teaspoons extra-virgin olive oil

Cauliflower Rice

DAIRY-FREE | GRAIN-FREE | NUT-FREE | VEGAN | UNDER 30 MINUTES

Cauliflower has a firm texture that makes it a suitable stand-in for rice when you are avoiding eating processed grains. It's super easy to make—almost easier than rice itself—and allows you to have a vegetable-forward meal with little fuss. **SERVES 4**

1. In a food processor or using a box grater, process the cauliflower until it is grated to the size of rice grains.

2. In a large skillet, heat the oil over medium heat. Add the cauliflower and stir well. Cover the skillet and steam the cauliflower for 5 to 7 minutes, until tender. Serve.

MAKE AHEAD If you find cauliflower on sale, buy a few heads and prepare them for meals throughout the week. Grate the cauliflower and pack into individual containers. Label how much is in each and freeze until ready to use. To cook, follow the directions in step 2, adding cooking time as needed to steam the cauliflower.

Per Serving: Calories: 68; Protein: 4g; Cholesterol: 0mg; Sodium: 63mg; Total Carbohydrates: 10g; Fiber: 4g; Total Fat: 2g; Saturated Fat: 0g

Roasted
Root Vegetable Medley

DAIRY-FREE | GRAIN-FREE | NUT-FREE | VEGAN

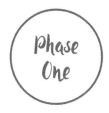

Phase One

This homey blend of root vegetables is a perfect diversion from the usual potato sides. Featuring a medley of sweet potato, carrots, beet, and onion and scented with rosemary, this simple mixture packs in so much big flavor that you won't even miss the starchy potato. It is a no-fuss side dish for every day. **SERVES 4**

PREP TIME: 10 MINUTES
COOK TIME: 40 MINUTES

1 large red onion, cut into wedges

2 large carrots, cut into 2-inch pieces

1 sweet potato, white or orange flesh, cut into 2-inch pieces

1 tablespoon extra-virgin olive oil, divided

1 large beet, peeled and cut into wedges

2 rosemary springs, stem removed and leaves roughly chopped

1. Preheat the oven to 400°F.

2. In a large bowl, toss the onion, carrots, and sweet potato with 2 teaspoons of olive oil.

3. In another bowl, toss the remaining 1 teaspoon of oil with the beet. Transfer the vegetables to a baking sheet and give it a shake so the vegetables settle in a single layer. Sprinkle with the rosemary.

4. Bake for 40 minutes, stirring the vegetables once halfway through. Serve.

INGREDIENT TIP Sweet potatoes are native to South America and come in many varieties, all of which have great nutritional value. Whether you select the orange-fleshed jewel or garnet varieties, or the light-colored Japanese versions, there is no need to peel the skin from a sweet potato before cooking. Because sweet potatoes are prone to spoilage, they should always be stored in a cool area.

Per Serving: Calories: 102; Protein: 2g; Cholesterol: 0mg; Sodium: 76mg; Total Carbohydrates: 17g; Fiber: 4g; Total Fat: 4g; Saturated Fat: 1g

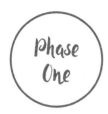

Phase One

PREP TIME: 10 MINUTES
COOK TIME: 22 MINUTES

1 pound Brussels sprouts, trimmed and halved

1 tablespoon extra-virgin olive oil

½ teaspoon salt

8 garlic cloves, minced

Juice of 1 lemon

Freshly ground black pepper

Roasted Garlic Brussels Sprouts

DAIRY-FREE | GRAIN-FREE | NUT-FREE | VEGAN

Roasting is a great way to cook vegetables because it allows you to get on with other things in the kitchen while they cook. And it also increases the sweetness of bitter vegetables like Brussels sprouts, making it the ideal cooking method for these little nutritional powerhouses. SERVES 4

1. Preheat the oven to 400°F.

2. In a large bowl, toss the Brussels sprouts, olive oil, and salt. Transfer them to a baking sheet and give it a shake so they settle in a single layer. Bake for 20 minutes, rotating the pan once halfway through.

3. Add the garlic to the baking sheet and cook for 2 minutes more. Remove from the oven, drizzle with the lemon juice, and toss. Season with pepper and more salt if desired. Serve.

Per Serving: Calories: 90; Protein: 4g; Cholesterol: 0mg; Sodium: 320mg; Total Carbohydrates: 13g; Fiber: 5g; Total Fat: 4g; Saturated Fat: 1g

Roasted Carrots with Goat Cheese

GRAIN-FREE | NUT-FREE | UNDER 30 MINUTES

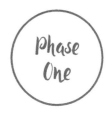

Roasting greatly enhances the sugars in carrots, making them an almost dessert-like treat. Here this simple masterpiece is topped with goat cheese to add a savory touch. **SERVES 4**

1. Preheat the oven to 400°F.

2. In a large bowl, toss the carrots with the garlic, olive oil, and thyme. Season with the salt and some pepper. Transfer the carrots to a baking sheet and give it a shake so they settle in a single layer. Bake for 15 to 20 minutes, stirring halfway through.

3. Transfer to a serving plate, top with the goat cheese, and serve.

Per Serving: Calories: 128; Protein: 3g; Cholesterol: 5mg; Sodium: 444mg; Total Carbohydrates: 17g; Fiber: 5g; Total Fat: 6g; Saturated Fat: 2g

PREP TIME: 5 MINUTES
COOK TIME: 20 MINUTES

1½ pounds carrots, halved lengthwise

3 garlic cloves, finely minced

1 tablespoon extra-virgin olive oil

½ teaspoon dried thyme

½ teaspoon salt

Freshly ground black pepper

¼ cup crumbled goat cheese

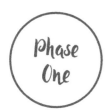

PREP TIME: 10 MINUTES
COOK TIME: 25 MINUTES

1 small sugar pumpkin, seeded and cut into wedges (see Tip)

6 to 8 garlic cloves, unpeeled

1 tablespoon extra-virgin olive oil

½ teaspoon salt

12 fresh sage leaves, for garnish

Baked Pumpkin with Garlic and Sage

DAIRY-FREE | GRAIN-FREE | NUT-FREE | VEGAN

Pumpkin is an underutilized vegetable in the kitchen, and that should change. Pumpkins are high in beta-carotene, as well as natural sugars, making them a satisfying treat any night of the week. SERVES 4

1. Preheat the oven to 400°F.

2. In a large bowl, toss the pumpkin with the garlic and olive oil. Season with the salt.

3. Bake for 20 to 25 minutes, until tender. Garnish with the sage leaves and serve.

SUBSTITUTION TIP Any type of winter squash can be roasted in this same way. Butternut, kabocha, delicata, and golden nugget squashes all roast really well and taste great.

Per Serving: Calories: 62; Protein: 1g; Cholesterol: 0mg; Sodium: 293mg; Total Carbohydrates: 8g; Fiber: 1g; Total Fat: 4g; Saturated Fat: 1g

Sautéed Collard Greens

DAIRY-FREE | GRAIN-FREE | NUT-FREE | UNDER 30 MINUTES | VEGAN

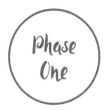

A member of the cabbage family, collards are unique for their large, tender leaves that are less bitter and slightly sweeter than other greens like kale. Collards are loaded with anticancer, antiviral, antioxidant, and antibiotic nutrients, making them about as close to medicine as you can get. Loaded with as much calcium as milk and plenty of soluble fiber, you may just want to eat them everyday, especially when as easily prepared as this recipe. SERVES 4

PREP TIME: 5 MINUTES
COOK TIME: 10 MINUTES

2 bunches collard greens, washed

2 teaspoons extra-virgin olive oil

Pinch red pepper flakes

½ teaspoon salt

Freshly ground black pepper

4 to 6 cloves garlic, minced

1. Place each collard green on a flat surface, folded with the stem facing out. Hold the leaf with one hand and use the other hand to pull the stem away from the leaf. Repeat with all the greens. Working in batches, stack the collards in a pile and slice into ½-inch strips.

2. In a large skillet, heat the oil over medium heat. Add the collards to the pan in batches, stirring as you add the greens. Continue stirring for 1 to 2 minutes, until the greens begin to wilt. Cover and reduce heat to medium-low, steaming the greens for about 5 minutes, stirring occasionally.

3. Remove the lid, and add the red pepper flakes, salt, pepper, and garlic. Stir for 1 to 2 additional minutes, until the garlic is fragrant and the greens tender. Serve.

Per Serving: Calories: 44; Protein: 2g; Cholesterol: 0mg; Sodium: 302mg; Total Carbohydrates: 5g; Fiber: 2g; Total Fat: 3g; Saturated Fat: 0g

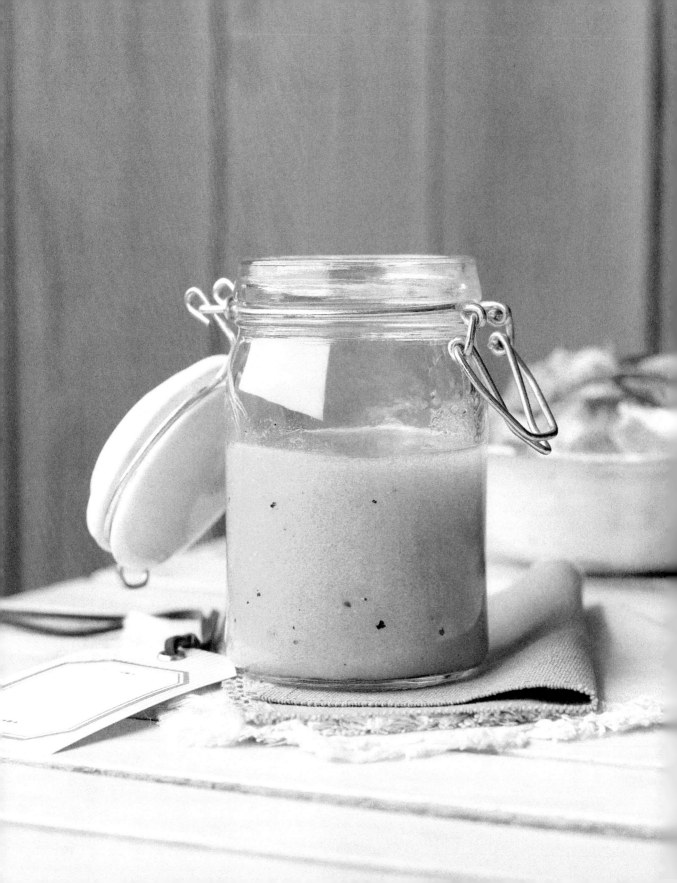

Homemade Basics, Sauces, and Condiments

Ditch the bottles of preservative- and sugar-laden dressings and sauces, and instead whip up a batch of these easy substitutes. Once you start to read labels, you will see that sugar is hiding in places you wouldn't expect—like tomato sauce and salad dressing. No need to worry though; this chapter has got you covered.

Taco Seasoning

DAIRY-FREE | GRAIN-FREE | NUT-FREE | VEGAN | UNDER 30 MINUTES

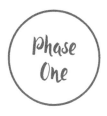

Phase One

Many store-bought taco seasonings contain stabilizers for thickening and preservatives to lengthen shelf life. However, you can easily avoid those unwanted additives by simply making this blend at home to have on hand when you need it. **MAKES ½ CUP**

In a small bowl, whisk the chili powder, cumin, garlic powder, paprika, onion powder, oregano, salt, and pepper to mix. Store in an airtight container for up to 6 months. Use 2 to 3 tablespoons of seasoning per 1 pound of meat or 2 cups of beans.

Per Serving (1 teaspoon): Calories: 4; Protein: 0g; Cholesterol: 0mg; Sodium: 60mg; Total Carbohydrates: 1g; Fiber: 0g; Total Fat: 0g; Saturated Fat: 0g

PREP TIME: 5 MINUTES

2 tablespoons chili powder

1 tablespoon ground cumin

2 teaspoons garlic powder

2 teaspoons ground paprika

2 teaspoons onion powder

1 teaspoon dried oregano

½ teaspoon salt

½ teaspoon freshly ground black pepper

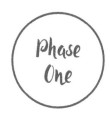

PREP TIME: 5 MINUTES
COOK TIME: 10 MINUTES

2 tablespoons extra-virgin olive oil

1 small yellow onion, finely chopped

1 garlic clove, minced

1 (28-ounce) can fire-roasted whole tomatoes

1 teaspoon dried basil

½ teaspoon dried oregano

Salt

Freshly ground black pepper

Tomato Marinara

DAIRY-FREE | GRAIN-FREE | NUT-FREE | VEGAN | UNDER 30 MINUTES

It's hard to find a commercial tomato sauce that is not sweetened with sugar or high-fructose corn syrup. Thankfully, a great-tasting tomato sauce like this one is really easy to make on your own. This recipe comes together in a matter of minutes, and you'll enjoy knowing it's additive-free. **MAKES ABOUT 1 QUART**

1. In a medium saucepan, heat the olive oil over medium heat. Sauté the onion and garlic until lightly browned, about 5 minutes.

2. Meanwhile, pour the tomatoes and their juices into a bowl and use your hands to break apart the tomatoes into smaller pieces.

3. Add the tomatoes to the saucepan and lower the heat to medium-low. Add the basil and oregano and simmer the sauce for 2 to 3 minutes.

4. Season with the salt and pepper. If a smoother sauce is preferred, purée the sauce in a blender or use an immersion blender. Serve hot.

Per Serving (½ cup): Calories: 66; Protein: 2g; Cholesterol: 0mg; Sodium: 151mg; Total Carbohydrates: 8g; Fiber: 2g; Total Fat: 4g; Saturated Fat: 1g

Ketchup

DAIRY-FREE | GRAIN-FREE | NUT-FREE | VEGAN | UNDER 30 MINUTES

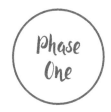

Ketchup is just one of many popular condiments that has become significantly sweeter over the years compared to its humble roots. More similar to early versions that were left unsweetened, this recipe uses a single date to add a little palatable sweetness while still being good for your gut. MAKES 1 CUP

In a blender, combine the tomatoes, soaked date, apple cider vinegar, salt, paprika, and onion powder. Process until smooth. Store in an airtight container in the refrigerator for up to 1 week.

DID YOU KNOW? Commercially canned tomatoes, like many other canned products, are very high in salt. When available, always choose low-sodium varieties of canned tomatoes.

Per Serving (2 tablespoons): Calories: 20; Protein: 0g; Cholesterol: 0mg; Sodium: 65mg; Total Carbohydrates: 4g; Fiber: 1g; Total Fat: 0g; Saturated Fat: 0g

PREP TIME: 5 MINUTES, PLUS 20 MINUTES SOAKING TIME

1 (15-ounce) can diced tomatoes, well drained and pressed in a colander to remove moisture

1 Medjool date, pitted and soaked in water for 20 minutes

1 teaspoon apple cider vinegar

Pinch salt

⅛ teaspoon paprika

¼ teaspoon onion powder

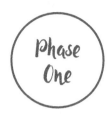

Phase One

PREP TIME: 15 MINUTES, PLUS OVERNIGHT TO REST
COOK TIME: 10 MINUTES, PLUS OVERNIGHT TO COMBINE

1¼ cups finely
   chopped cucumber
⅔ cup finely chopped
   yellow onion
⅔ cup finely chopped red
   bell pepper
1 garlic clove, finely minced
2 teaspoons salt
1 cup white vinegar
1 teaspoon yellow
   mustard seeds
½ teaspoon dill seeds
Pinch turmeric

Dill Relish

DAIRY-FREE | GRAIN-FREE | NUT-FREE | VEGAN

Store-bought relish is typically laden with sugar, but this recipe is not. This simple, tangy condiment can be prepped in minutes, and after an overnight rest, it can be finished in 10 minutes. A day later, giving time for the flavors to blend, it's ready to slather on burgers and patties. **MAKES 2 CUPS**

1. In a medium bowl, mix the cucumber, onion, bell pepper, and garlic. Toss with the salt and fill the bowl with water to cover the vegetables. Cover with a clean kitchen towel and leave the bowl to rest at room temperature for at least 6 hours or overnight. This will help expel excess water from the vegetables.

2. Drain the vegetables, rinse them with water, and drain again.

3. In a saucepan over medium heat, combine the vinegar, mustard seeds, dill seeds, and turmeric. Bring to a simmer and add the drained cucumber mixture. Reduce the heat to medium-low and simmer, uncovered, for 10 minutes.

4. Transfer to a pint jar, cover with an airtight lid, and let it rest until it is cool to the touch. Transfer to the refrigerator and let sit for at least 24 hours before serving. The relish will keep in the refrigerator for up to 1 month.

Per Serving (2 tablespoons): Calories: 9; Protein: 0g; Cholesterol: 0mg; Sodium: 292mg; Total Carbohydrates: 1g; Fiber: 0g; Total Fat: 0g; Saturated Fat: 0g

Red Wine Vinaigrette

DAIRY-FREE | GRAIN-FREE | NUT-FREE | VEGAN | UNDER 30 MINUTES

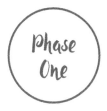

Phase One

Red wine vinaigrette is one of the most universally useful dressings you can make. It tastes just as good on a simple salad as it does on a quinoa bowl and comes together in minutes. **MAKES ½ CUP**

PREP TIME: 5 MINUTES

In a small bowl, whisk the vinegar, mustard, salt, and pepper together. Pour the olive oil into the bowl in a steady stream while whisking until thoroughly mixed. The vinaigrette can be stored, tightly covered, in the refrigerator for 1 to 2 days.

- 3 tablespoons red wine vinegar
- 1 teaspoon Dijon mustard
- ¼ teaspoon salt
- ¼ teaspoon freshly ground black pepper
- ⅓ cup extra-virgin olive oil

Per Serving (2 tablespoons): Calories: 162; Protein: 0g; Cholesterol: 0mg; Sodium: 177mg; Total Carbohydrates: 0g; Fiber: 0g; Total Fat: 18g; Saturated Fat: 2.5g

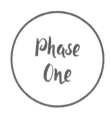

Phase
One

PREP TIME: 5 MINUTES

¼ cup freshly squeezed
   lemon juice

1 teaspoon freshly grated
   lemon zest

5 garlic cloves, minced

¼ cup extra-virgin olive oil

1 teaspoon salt

½ teaspoon freshly ground
   black pepper

Bright Lemon-Garlic Vinaigrette

DAIRY-FREE | GRAIN-FREE | NUT-FREE | VEGAN | UNDER 30 MINUTES

This vibrant vinaigrette brightens just about anything it touches. Drizzle it over salad greens or add it to a quinoa bowl, and you have a delicious dish with a gourmet feel in little time. **MAKES ½ CUP**

In a small bowl, whisk the lemon juice, lemon zest, garlic, and olive oil. Season with the salt and pepper. The vinaigrette can be stored, tightly covered, in the refrigerator for 1 to 2 days.

Per Serving (2 tablespoons): Calories: 128; Protein: 0g; Cholesterol: 0mg; Sodium: 292mg; Total Carbohydrates: 2g; Fiber: 0g; Total Fat: 14g; Saturated Fat: 2g

Mustard Vinaigrette

DAIRY-FREE | GRAIN-FREE | NUT-FREE | VEGAN | UNDER 30 MINUTES

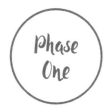

Mustard may seem like an unlikely ingredient in a dressing, but its bold, robust flavor actually tastes really good with just about any kind of greens. Use a good-quality raw apple cider vinegar for the most health benefits. **MAKES ½ CUP**

In a small bowl, whisk together the apple cider vinegar, mustard, olive oil, and garlic. Season with the salt and some pepper. The vinaigrette can be stored, tightly covered, in the refrigerator for 1 to 2 days.

Per Serving (2 tablespoons): Calories: 124; Protein: 0g; Cholesterol: 0mg; Sodium: 236mg; Total Carbohydrates: 1g; Fiber: 0g; Total Fat: 14g; Saturated Fat: 2g

PREP TIME: 5 MINUTES

3 tablespoons apple
cider vinegar

1 tablespoon Dijon mustard

¼ cup extra-virgin olive oil

1 garlic clove, finely minced

¼ teaspoon salt

Freshly ground
black pepper

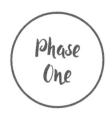

PREP TIME: 5 MINUTES

¼ cup unsweetened
plain yogurt

¼ cup unsweetened plain
almond milk

½ cup crumbled
blue cheese

Juice of 1 lemon

¼ teaspoon salt

¼ teaspoon freshly ground
black pepper

Blue Cheese Dressing

GRAIN-FREE | NUT-FREE | UNDER 30 MINUTES

This savory and funky favorite cuts out the traditional
high-in-fat mayonnaise, sour cream, and cream by
using yogurt and almond milk for a probiotic dressing
that is big on flavor. **MAKES 1 CUP**

In a small bowl, whisk together the yogurt and almond milk.
Add the blue cheese and lemon juice, and stir to combine. Season with the salt and pepper. The dressing can be stored, tightly
covered, in the refrigerator for up to 3 days.

Per Serving (2 tablespoons): Calories: 42; Protein: 3g; Cholesterol: 9mg;
Sodium: 205mg; Total Carbohydrates: 2g; Fiber: 0g; Total Fat: 3g; Saturated Fat: 2g

Skinny Caesar Dressing

GRAIN-FREE | NUT-FREE

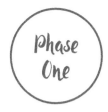

The backbone of that true Caesar salad flavor is anchovy. The unique flavor of the fish is what ties the dressing together, so be sure to use it. **MAKES ½ CUP**

In a blender, combine the anchovy, garlic, yogurt, almond milk, lemon juice, mustard, and Worcestershire sauce and process until smooth. Let rest for 1 hour, or preferably overnight, before using to allow the flavors to meld. The finished dressing can be stored, tightly covered, in the refrigerator for 2 to 3 days.

Per Serving (2 tablespoons): Calories: 28; Protein: 2g; Cholesterol: 5mg; Sodium: 105mg; Total Carbohydrates: 3g; Fiber: 0g; Total Fat: 1g; Saturated Fat: 1g

PREP TIME: 5 MINUTES, PLUS 1 HOUR TO REST

1 anchovy fillet

1 garlic clove

½ cup unsweetened plain yogurt

2 tablespoons unsweetened plain almond milk

1 tablespoon freshly squeezed lemon juice

1 teaspoon Dijon mustard

1 teaspoon Worcestershire sauce

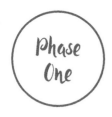

PREP TIME: 5 MINUTES

2 tablespoons tahini

1 garlic clove, finely minced

½ cup unsweetened
plain yogurt

3 tablespoons extra-virgin
olive oil

Juice of 1 lemon

¼ teaspoon salt

¼ teaspoon freshly ground
black pepper

Yogurt Tahini Dressing

GRAIN-FREE | NUT-FREE | UNDER 30 MINUTES

Tahini, the ground paste of sesame seeds, is a powerful base for a dressing. With a strong sesame flavor, this simple dressing can top a salad, fish, or poultry for a savory combination that shines. **MAKES ¾ CUP**

1. In a small bowl, whisk the tahini and 2 tablespoons hot water together until a smooth paste is formed.

2. Add the garlic, yogurt, olive oil, and lemon juice and stir to combine. Season with the salt and pepper. The finished dressing can be stored, tightly covered, in the refrigerator for up to 3 days.

Per Serving (2 tablespoons): Calories: 105; Protein: 2g; Cholesterol: 3mg; Sodium: 116mg; Total Carbohydrates: 3g; Fiber: 1g; Total Fat: 10g; Saturated Fat: 2g

Herbed Olive Oil

DAIRY-FREE | GRAIN-FREE | NUT-FREE | VEGAN

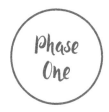

Phase One

With three-quarters of its fat content being the heart-healthy monounsaturated variety, olive oil is a good fat that you should consume regularly. This simple herbed oil will brighten steamed vegetables, liven fish, or even complement a baked potato. Use any extra herbs you have lying around your kitchen to make this oil before they go bad, and give them new life in this flavorful condiment that is a must-have in your kitchen. **MAKES 1 CUP**

PREP TIME: 5 MINUTES
COOK TIME: 5 MINUTES, PLUS 2 HOUR REST

1 cup extra-virgin olive oil
5 garlic cloves, crushed
¼ cup parsley leaves
¼ cup basil leaves
2 to 3 thyme sprigs
¼ teaspoon black peppercorns

1. In a small saucepan, heat the oil over low heat until warmed, but not smoking.

2. Place the garlic, parsley, basil, thyme, and peppercorns in a bowl, then add the heated oil. Let rest for 2 hours.

3. Place a wire mesh strainer over a jar, and pour the oil into the jar, straining out the herbs. Use immediately.

Per Serving (1 tablespoon): Calories: 41; Protein: 0g; Cholesterol: 0mg; Sodium: 1mg; Total Carbohydrates: 0g; Fiber: 0g; Total Fat: 5g; Saturated Fat: 1g

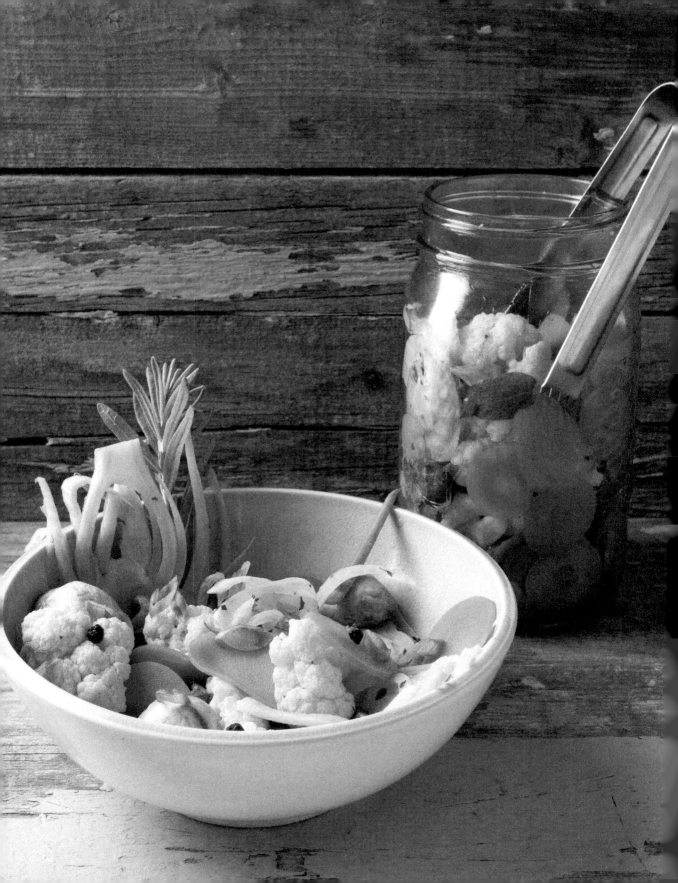

Easy Ferments

Fermenting foods yourself is a good way to lower your grocery bills. These simple ferments are easy to get right and are actually fun to make. In just a few steps you can transform ordinary vegetables, fruits, and dairy into probiotic products that can help support your gut health; you will be happy you took the leap.

« *Fermented Cauliflower, Carrots, and Red Onions* (page 215)

Kefir

GRAIN-FREE | NUT-FREE

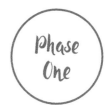

PREP TIME: 5 MINUTES
FERMENTATION TIME: 24 HOURS

Kefir is one of the easiest dairy ferments to make and can be used in a variety of ways to add a probiotic punch to your diet. Serve it with granola or blend it with fruit and drink it. Use it in baking as a low-lactose replacement for milk or yogurt, or blend it into soups after cooking for a creamy probiotic edge. It is extremely versatile, quite affordable when made at home, and easy to keep going indefinitely once you get into a regular rhythm. **MAKES 2 CUPS**

2 cups whole milk

1 tablespoon hydrated kefir grains

1. In a pint jar, combine the milk and kefir grains. Cover the jar with a clean kitchen towel secured by a rubber band and place in a room-temperature location for 24 hours.

2. Place a funnel inside another pint jar. Pour the liquid through a fine-mesh strainer into the funnel. Tap the strainer gently against the funnel so that all the liquid drains into the jar below, leaving just the grains. Cover the kefir with a tight-fitting lid and refrigerate for up to 5 days. The grains may be transferred into a third jar and covered with another 2 cups whole milk to begin the process again for your next batch.

DID YOU KNOW? Kefir grains can be purchased online if they are not available locally. Choose the slightly more expensive grains over the ready-set powder when possible. The grains last indefinitely when taken care of, and require no heating of the milk, which will save you time. Be sure to follow the package instructions regarding rehydrating the grains before using.

Per Serving (1 cup): Calories: 160; Protein: 8g; Cholesterol: 30mg; Sodium: 125mg; Total Carbohydrates: 12g; Fiber: 0g; Total Fat: 8g; Saturated Fat: 5g

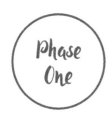

Phase One

PREP TIME: 10 MINUTES,
PLUS 30 MINUTES TO REST
FERMENTATION TIME:
3 TO 14 DAYS

1 (2- to 3-pound) head
red cabbage
1½ tablespoons sea salt

Sauerkraut

DAIRY-FREE | GRAIN-FREE | NUT-FREE | VEGAN

Sauerkraut takes the prize as the easiest vegetable ferment to make at home, and when you make it yourself, you can skip the pricey artisanal versions popping up in stores nationwide. Buy a head of cabbage and embark on this easy project for just a few dollars and minutes of your time. Because of its nice bright color and unbeatable vitamin profile, I recommend red cabbage, but you can easily swap it for green if needed. **MAKES 1 QUART**

1. Discard the outer leaves of the cabbage and cut the cabbage in half through its core. Remove the core and slice each half lengthwise into thin ribbons about ¼ inch thick.

2. In a large bowl, toss the cabbage with the salt. Leave it to sit at room temperature for 30 minutes.

3. Transfer the cabbage to a quart jar, packing it down firmly with your fist or a kitchen tool as needed. Pour any juices from the bowl into the jar and again press the cabbage down firmly.

4. Cover the jar loosely with a lid and leave it at room temperature. After 24 hours, the brine should cover the cabbage. If not, mix 1 teaspoon of salt with 1 cup of water and pour this over the cabbage until it is submerged. Use a weight to hold the cabbage below the brine and loosely cover the jar with a lid.

5. Ferment at room temperature for 3 to 14 days. After 3 days, begin tasting it. When it is to your liking, remove the weight and transfer the sauerkraut to the refrigerator where it will keep for several months.

DID YOU KNOW? Lactic acid fermentation is an anaerobic process, meaning it takes place in the absence of oxygen. For this reason, it is important to keep fermenting foods below the brine for the process to work correctly. To do this, a small jelly jar, glass votive candleholder, or even a rock can be used to weight the food below the surface of the brine. To prevent spoilage, just be sure that whatever you use is cleaned and sanitized before adding to your food.

Per Serving (2 tablespoons): Calories: 6; Protein: 0g; Cholesterol: 0mg; Sodium: 332mg; Total Carbohydrates: 1g; Fiber: 1g; Total Fat: 0g; Saturated Fat: 0g

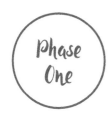

PREP TIME: 10 MINUTES
FERMENTATION TIME:
3 DAYS TO 2 WEEKS

3½ tablespoons sea
  salt, divided

2 pounds napa
  cabbage, cut into 1- to
  2-inch squares

1 small carrot, sliced on
  the diagonal

4 scallions, white and
  green parts, cut on
  the diagonal into
  2-inch pieces

6 garlic cloves, crushed

1 (2-inch) piece
  fresh ginger, cut
  into matchsticks

1½ tablespoons Korean
  ground red pepper

Sesame seeds, for serving

Kimchi with Sesame Seeds

DAIRY-FREE | GRAIN-FREE | NUT-FREE | VEGAN

Kimchi is the spicy, funky cousin of sauerkraut. Loaded with ginger and Korean chili powder, this easy probiotic pickle is a powerhouse condiment that tastes great with whole grains. **MAKES 1 QUART**

1. In a large bowl, dissolve 3 tablespoons of salt in 4 cups of water.

2. Add the cabbage and carrot. Cover with a plate to hold the vegetables below the brine and then cover the bowl with a clean kitchen towel. Let it sit overnight at room temperature.

3. The following day, strain the brine from the vegetables into a bowl set under a colander. Set the brine aside and return the vegetables to the bowl in which they were brined.

4. Mix the scallions, garlic, ginger, Korean pepper, and remaining 1½ teaspoons of salt into the cabbage and stir well to combine. Pack the mixture into a quart jar, pressing down firmly as you pack the jar, leaving a 1-inch headspace. Fill any remaining space in the jar with the reserved brine so that the vegetables are covered. If needed, use a small weight to hold the vegetables below the brine. Cover lightly with a lid and leave to ferment in a cool location, around 68°F.

5. Ferment for 3 days, loosening the lid daily to release gases. Taste the kimchi, and if it is adequately soured, replace the lid tightly and transfer the jar to the refrigerator. If not, continue to ferment for up to 2 weeks until it is to your liking. There is no right or wrong timeline for kimchi. Use your taste buds to determine what is right for you.

6. Serve, sprinkled with sesame seeds. The kimchi will keep in the refrigerator for 1 month.

Per Serving (2 tablespoons): Calories: 10; Protein: 0g; Cholesterol: 0mg; Sodium: 781mg; Total Carbohydrates: 2g; Fiber: 0g; Total Fat: 0g; Saturated Fat: 0g

Fermented Cauliflower, Carrots, and Red Onions

DAIRY-FREE | GRAIN-FREE | NUT-FREE | VEGAN

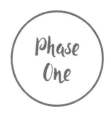

Antipasto plates have never been better than with this simple fermented vegetable mixture. Make the medley using the simpler method below, or add your favorite whole spices such as cumin, fennel, anise, caraway, or dill for your own unique twist on this classic fermented pickle. MAKES 1 QUART

PREP TIME: 10 MINUTES
FERMENTATION TIME:
5 TO 7 DAYS

2 tablespoons sea salt

2 cups cauliflower florets, broken into small pieces

2 carrots, sliced on the diagonal

1 red onion, cut into wedges

1 small hot chile

1. In a bowl, dissolve the salt in 4 cups of water and set it aside.

2. Pack the cauliflower, carrots, onion, and chile into a quart jar. Pour the brine over the vegetables, using a small weight to keep the vegetables submerged if needed, and cover the jar loosely with a lid. Leave to ferment in a room-temperature location.

3. Ferment for 5 to 7 days. After 2 days, begin opening the lid daily to release built-up gases. When the vegetables are fermented to your liking, remove the weight, replace the lid tightly, and transfer to the refrigerator, where they will keep for several months.

Per Serving (¼ cup): Calories: 9; Protein: 1g; Cholesterol: 0mg; Sodium: 895mg; Total Carbohydrates: 2g; Fiber: 1g; Total Fat: 0g; Saturated Fat: 0g

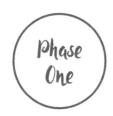

PREP TIME: 10 MINUTES
FERMENTATION TIME: 2 DAYS

1½ tablespoons sea salt
1 pound carrots, cut
   into sticks

Fermented Carrot Sticks

DAIRY-FREE | GRAIN-FREE | NUT-FREE | VEGAN

If you are going to snack on carrots, why not add a few probiotics to the mix? These simple carrot sticks are bursting with an unexpected tangy flavor and will have you reaching for more. Serve them on their own or with Eggplant Yogurt Dip (page 179) for even more flavor. **MAKES 1 QUART**

1. In a large jar, dissolve the salt in 2 cups of water.

2. Pack the carrots tightly into the jar so that they are held in place, and leave about 1 inch of headspace. If necessary, use a weight to hold the carrots below the brine.

3. Cover loosely with a lid and leave to ferment at room temperature for 2 to 3 days, until you like the flavor of the carrots. Open the jar once a day to release gases.

4. Cover tightly with a lid and transfer to the refrigerator where the carrots will improve with age. Store for up to 2 weeks.

DID YOU KNOW? A narrow-mouth quart jar works well for a ferment such as carrots, as the mouth of the jar can actually be used to hold the carrots in place below the brine. Pack the carrots tightly and cover with brine. Ensure that none are floating before covering the jar. If necessary, pack more carrot spears into the jar to hold them in place.

Per Serving (2 or 3 sticks): Calories: 12; Protein: 0g; Cholesterol: 0mg; Sodium: 683mg; Total Carbohydrates: 3g; Fiber: 1g; Total Fat: 0g; Saturated Fat: 0g

Fermented Salsa

DAIRY-FREE | GRAIN-FREE | NUT-FREE | VEGAN

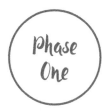

Salsa is one of those foods that is so great to serve before a meal, it is hard to believe that it can get any better. But it can. Enter the fermented version. This simple blend of tomatoes, onion, and jalapeño is transformed into a masterpiece with a 48-hour fermentation. **MAKES 1 QUART**

PREP TIME: 10 MINUTES
FERMENTATION TIME:
48 HOURS

1 small yellow onion, diced

2 large tomatoes, diced

1 jalapeño pepper, diced

1 garlic clove, minced

¼ cup chopped
   fresh cilantro

Juice of 1 lime

2 teaspoons sea salt

1. In a small bowl, toss the onion, tomatoes, jalapeño, garlic, and cilantro. Add the lime juice and salt, and mix well.

2. Transfer the salsa to a quart jar and press the vegetables down lightly so that the juice covers them. Cover loosely with a lid and leave to ferment at room temperature for 48 hours.

3. Close the lid tightly and transfer to the refrigerator, where the salsa can be stored for up to 10 days.

Per Serving (½ cup): Calories: 40; Protein: 2g; Cholesterol: 0mg; Sodium: 596mg; Total Carbohydrates: 9g; Fiber: 1g; Total Fat: 0g; Saturated Fat: 0g

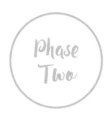

Phase Two

PREP TIME: 5 MINUTES
COOK TIME: 5 MINUTES
FERMENTATION TIME:
48 HOURS

2 pints fresh raspberries
2 tablespoons honey
¾ teaspoon sea salt
2 tablespoons whey
¼ cup chia seeds

Fermented Raspberry Chia Jam

GRAIN-FREE | NUT-FREE

Making jam has never been easier than it is with chia seeds. These gelatinous powerhouses allow for a quick-cook jam with the perfect spreadable consistency. Locking in plenty of probiotics, this jam is excellent spooned over yogurt, muesli, or granola. **MAKES 1 PINT**

1. In a small saucepan, heat the raspberries over low heat, mashing them gently with a fork to release their juices. Simmer for 5 minutes, until they are broken down well. Remove the saucepan from the heat and let the raspberries cool for a few minutes.

2. Add the honey and salt to the raspberries and stir well. Transfer the jam to a pint jar and cover loosely.

3. Once cool to the touch, add the whey and chia seeds, and stir to incorporate. Cover loosely with a lid and leave to ferment at room temperature for 48 hours. Open the jar once daily to release excess gases.

4. Close the lid tightly and transfer to the refrigerator, where the jam will keep for several weeks.

DID YOU KNOW? When fermenting, it is important to use salt that is free of additives. Sea salt, pickling salt, and canning salt are great choices for fermentation.

DID YOU KNOW? Whey is a by-product of dairy fermentation, often discarded at the end of the process of cheesemaking. To make your own, line a colander with several layers of cheesecloth and strain unsweetened plain yogurt or kefir over a bowl. The liquid extracted is whey. Refrigerate it in an airtight container for up to 1 month.

Per Serving (2 tablespoons): Calories: 47; Protein: 1g; Cholesterol: 0mg; Sodium: 113mg; Total Carbohydrates: 9g; Fiber: 4g; Total Fat: 1g; Saturated Fat: 0g

Fermented Cranberry Sauce

GRAIN-FREE | NUT-FREE

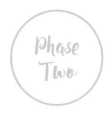

Phase Two

If you have only had the stuff out of a can, you have got to try this! This salty, sweet, and sour blend is delicious. Bursting with cinnamon, it can transform a turkey meal or simply be eaten by the spoonful. Serve it alongside meat dishes, mix some into a bowl of yogurt, or add it to a smoothie for a special treat. **SERVES 16**

PREP TIME: 5 MINUTES
FERMENTATION TIME: 48 HOURS

1 (12-ounce) bag cranberries

½ cup honey

1 teaspoon non-iodized salt

½ cup whey

1 teaspoon ground cinnamon

Juice of 2 oranges

Juice of 1 lemon

½ cup golden raisins

1. In a blender, combine the cranberries, honey, salt, whey, cinnamon, orange juice, and lemon juice. Process briefly, until still slightly chunky.

2. Transfer to a quart jar and cover with a lid, tightening just barely. Leave the jar at room temperature for 48 hours.

3. Mix in the raisins, close the lid tightly, and transfer the sauce to the refrigerator. Store for up to 1 month.

INGREDIENT TIP Cranberries are typically only available at the store around the holidays. However, they can be easily frozen in the same bag they are sold in. Simply pop the bag in the freezer until needed.

Per Serving: Calories: 65; Protein: 0g; Cholesterol: 0mg; Sodium: 153mg; Total Carbohydrates: 17g; Fiber: 1g; Total Fat: 0g; Saturated Fat: 0g

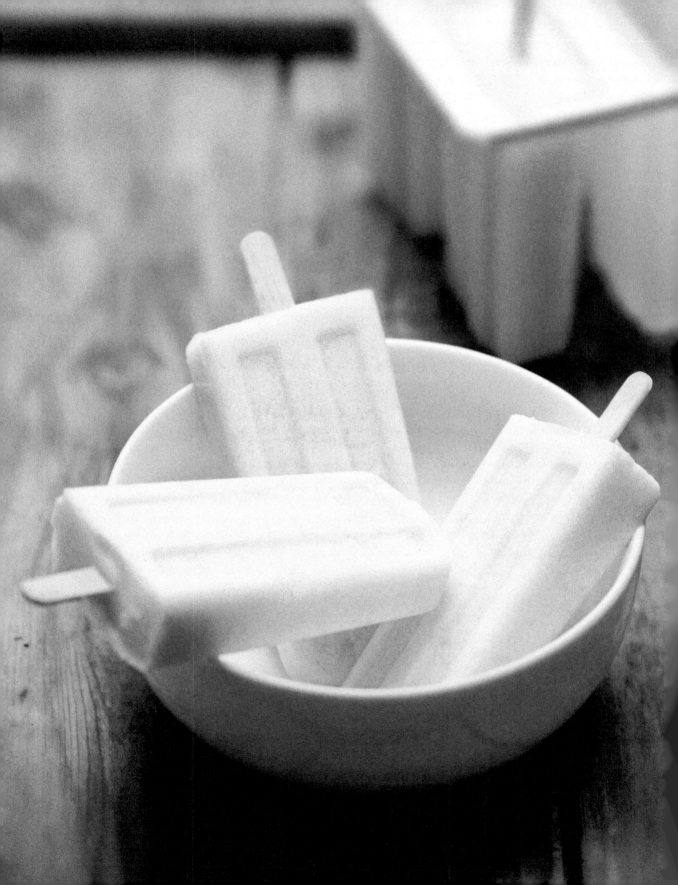

Desserts

Just because sugar is limited on the microbiome diet, it doesn't mean that you are not able to indulge in dessert. These desserts all rely on the original sweet food: fruit. Loaded with natural sugars, fruits take the starring roles in these treats to add flavor and satisfy your sweet tooth. Surprisingly, after a couple of weeks on the microbiome diet, you may find yourself reaching for these simple fruit-infused desserts instead of the sugary and fatty treats you used to crave.

Cantaloupe Mint Granita

DAIRY-FREE | GRAIN-FREE | NUT-FREE | VEGAN

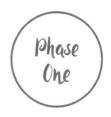

A granita is a lovely frozen treat. They are often sugar bombs, but this fruit-forward preparation will satisfy your sweet tooth and keep your body in check. The mint infusion comes together while you cut the cantaloupe, adding a bright tone to the melon and producing gourmet results. SERVES 4

PREP TIME: 10 MINUTES, PLUS 30 MINUTES TO FREEZE

¼ cup fresh mint leaves
1 cantaloupe, halved
  and seeded

1. In a small saucepan over medium-high heat, combine the mint leaves and 1 cup of water. Bring to a boil, reduce the heat to low, and simmer for 5 minutes, reducing the liquid by half.

2. Meanwhile, remove the flesh from the cantaloupe and transfer it to a blender. Process until smooth.

3. Strain the mint water, discarding the mint leaves. Add the mint-infused water to the blender with the cantaloupe and process until thoroughly incorporated.

4. Transfer the cantaloupe mixture to a 9-by-9-inch baking dish and place it in the freezer for 15 minutes. Using a fork, break up the mixture and then place it back in the freezer for 15 more minutes. Again, break up the now nearly frozen mixture into small pieces. Serve.

MAKE AHEAD This can be made ahead but tends to freeze pretty solid if left unstirred. Remove from the freezer about 10 minutes before serving and use a fork to break up the granita.

Per Serving: Calories: 47; Protein: 1g; Cholesterol: 0mg; Sodium: 22mg; Total Carbohydrates: 11g; Fiber: 1g; Total Fat: 0g; Saturated Fat: 0g

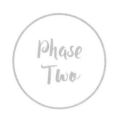

Phase Two

PREP TIME: 5 MINUTES, PLUS 2 HOURS TO FREEZE

¼ cup honey

1 pound strawberries, hulled

2 teaspoons pure vanilla extract

Strawberry Vanilla Sorbet

DAIRY-FREE | GRAIN-FREE | NUT-FREE

Sorbet is a frozen dessert made using puréed fruit and a simple syrup. This variation is great in the early summer when fresh local strawberries are abundant, but it can also be made with frozen packaged strawberries. Honey and vanilla boost the flavor while still keeping the treat lower in overall sugar than commercial sorbet varieties. **SERVES 4**

1. In a microwave-safe dish, combine the honey and ¼ cup water. Microwave for 20 to 30 seconds, until just warm, and stir to mix the two together.

2. In a blender, combine the strawberries, honey mixture, and vanilla. Process until smooth.

3. Pour into a 9-by-9-inch baking dish and freeze until firm, about 2 hours.

4. To serve, transfer the sorbet to the blender and process until smooth.

SUBSTITUTION TIP This can be made using any type of soft fruit that you like. Some great ones to try are honeydew, all types of berries, and peaches.

Per Serving: Calories: 107; Protein: 0g; Cholesterol: 0mg; Sodium: 2mg; Total Carbohydrates: 26g; Fiber: 2g; Total Fat: 0g; Saturated Fat: 0g

Grilled Peaches *and* Vanilla Yogurt

GRAIN-FREE | NUT-FREE | UNDER 30 MINUTES

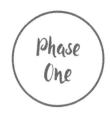

Phase One

PREP TIME: 5 MINUTES
COOK TIME: 10 MINUTES

Grilling peaches caramelizes the sugar of the fruit and creates a stunningly simple and delicious dessert. When paired with vanilla yogurt, this low-sugar dessert is a wonderful treat that can be enjoyed in both phases of the microbiome diet. **SERVES 2**

1 cup unsweetened plain low-fat yogurt

1 teaspoon pure vanilla extract

1 peach, halved and pitted

1. In a small bowl, mix the yogurt and vanilla together. Divide between two bowls.

2. Heat a grill or grill pan to high and lightly oil the grate.

3. Place the peach halves, cut-side down, on the grill and cook for 3 to 5 minutes, until the cut surface is well browned. Flip and continue to cook for 1 to 2 minutes more, until heated through.

4. Top each bowl of yogurt with a half peach and serve.

SUBSTITUTION TIP Stone fruits are great for grilling. Consider using another variety such as nectarine or plum, which both hold up well when grilled. Pineapple also works well when prepared in this way.

Per Serving: Calories: 115; Protein: 5g; Cholesterol: 18mg; Sodium: 75mg; Total Carbohydrates: 14g; Fiber: 1g; Total Fat: 4g; Saturated Fat: 3g

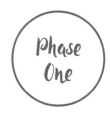

Phase One

PREP TIME: 5 MINUTES, PLUS 5 TO 6 HOURS TO FREEZE

2 tablespoons coconut cream

3 cups frozen pineapple chunks

1 teaspoon pure vanilla extract

Pineapple Coconut Ice Pops

DAIRY-FREE | GRAIN-FREE | NUT-FREE | VEGAN

If you want to feel as if you are on the beach in the Caribbean, these ice pops will do the trick. Using no added sugar, these icy treats pack a lot of flavor into their small forms. Using frozen pineapple, these will freeze quickly. A fresh pineapple can be used instead, but you will have to adjust the freezing time accordingly. **SERVES 8**

1. In a blender, combine the coconut cream and ¾ cup of water and process until smooth. Add the pineapple and vanilla, and process until smooth. Pour the mixture into 8 ice-pop molds.

2. Freeze until solid, 5 to 6 hours. Serve.

Per Serving: Calories: 45; Protein: 1g; Cholesterol: 0mg; Sodium: 1mg; Total Carbohydrates: 8g; Fiber: 1g; Total Fat: 1g; Saturated Fat: 1g

Honey-Berry Yogurt Ice Pops

GRAIN-FREE | NUT-FREE

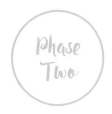

Phase Two

Popsicles are a lovely and refreshing treat. These simple fruit pops will satisfy your sweet tooth and are much better for you than store-bought varieties, which are typically laden with sugars and corn syrup. If you don't have an ice-pop mold, use small paper cups and wooden treat sticks to make your own. SERVES 8

1. In a blender, combine the yogurt, blueberries, raspberries, and honey and process until smooth. Pour into 8 ice-pop molds.

2. Freeze until solid, 5 to 6 hours. Serve.

SUBSTITUTION TIP Make these simple freezer pops with any of your favorite fruits; just be sure to use about 2 cups of fruit for every 2 cups of yogurt.

Per Serving: Calories: 82; Protein: 3g; Cholesterol: 9mg; Sodium: 38mg; Total Carbohydrates: 15g; Fiber: 2g; Total Fat: 2g; Saturated Fat: 1g

PREP TIME: 5 MINUTES, PLUS 5 TO 6 HOURS TO FREEZE

2 cups unsweetened plain low-fat yogurt

1 cup blueberries

1 cup raspberries

3 tablespoons honey

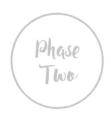

PREP TIME: 5 MINUTES
COOK TIME: 20 MINUTES

FOR THE CRÊPES

4 eggs

¾ cup almond flour

1 tablespoon canola oil,
  plus more for the pan

¾ cup unsweetened plain
  almond milk

Pinch salt

FOR THE FILLING

1 cup raspberries

1 cup blueberries

2 tablespoons honey

Juice of 1 lemon

Almond Flour Crêpes with Mixed Berry Filling

DAIRY-FREE | GRAIN-FREE | UNDER 30 MINUTES

The traditional thin French pancake gets a gluten-free makeover in this almond-flour remake. Filled with a blueberry-raspberry sauce, these crêpes are a must-try, especially when you want something rich and warm. **SERVES 6**

TO MAKE THE CRÊPES

1. In a blender, combine the eggs, almond flour, 1 tablespoon of canola oil, the almond milk, and salt. Process until the batter is smooth, scraping down the sides of the blender as needed.

2. In a large skillet over medium-low heat, add just enough oil to lightly coat the pan and heat until just shimmering.

3. Add a scant ¼ cup of batter to the pan. Use the back of a spoon to swirl the batter over the entire surface of the skillet so that it reaches all the way to the edges.

4. When the edges become set, use a spatula to loosen the crêpe all the way around the skillet. Flip the crêpe and continue to cook for 1 to 2 minutes more, until light brown and set. Transfer the crêpe to a plate and continue to make more crêpes using the rest of the batter. Lay a sheet of parchment paper between each crêpe to keep them separated as they come out of the skillet.

TO MAKE THE FILLING

1. In a medium saucepan, heat the raspberries, blueberries, honey, and lemon juice over medium-high heat. Cook for about 5 minutes, gently stirring the berries until they begin to release their juices and soften. Remove from the heat.

2. Spoon equal amounts of the fruit filling into the center of each crêpe and fold the crêpe over to enclose the filling. Serve.

Per Serving: Calories: 289; Protein: 11g; Cholesterol: 139mg; Sodium: 102mg; Total Carbohydrates: 19g; Fiber: 5g; Total Fat: 21g; Saturated Fat: 2g

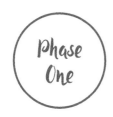

Phase One

Juice of 4 limes

¼ cup chia seeds

Freshly grated zest of 2 limes

2 teaspoons pure vanilla extract

2 Medjool dates, pitted

1 frozen banana

1 cup baby spinach

2 cups unsweetened plain almond milk

Lime-Chia Smoothie

DAIRY-FREE | GRAIN-FREE | VEGAN | UNDER 30 MINUTES

This dessert smoothie is similar to a limeade and is wholeheartedly refreshing. Chia seeds boost the fiber, making it an even better dessert choice. **SERVES 2**

1. In a small bowl, combine the lime juice and chia seeds, and let it sit for 20 minutes, until the seeds swell.

2. In a blender, combine the lime-chia mixture, lime zest, vanilla, dates, banana, spinach, and almond milk. Process until smooth and serve.

Per Serving: Calories: 343; Protein: 8g; Cholesterol: 0mg; Sodium: 200mg; Total Carbohydrates: 55g; Fiber: 16g; Total Fat: 13g; Saturated Fat: 1g

Cinnamon Rice Pudding

DAIRY-FREE

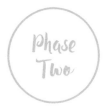

Phase Two

Loaded with warming cinnamon, this is a great winter dessert that hits the spot. Raisins and honey add sweetness, while almond extract gives the pudding a nutty, savory flavor. **SERVES 4**

PREP TIME: 5 MINUTES
COOK TIME: 1 HOUR

1. In a small saucepan over medium-high heat, combine the brown rice, salt, and 2 cups of water. Bring to a boil, reduce the heat to low, cover, and simmer for about 45 minutes, until all the water has been absorbed.

2. Add the almond milk, raisins, almond extract, honey, and cinnamon. Bring to a simmer and continue to cook for 15 minutes more, stirring frequently, until creamy.

1 cup brown rice

¼ teaspoon salt

¾ cup unsweetened plain almond milk

2 tablespoons golden raisins

¼ teaspoon almond extract

3 tablespoons honey

1 teaspoon ground cinnamon

DID YOU KNOW? Golden raisins are made from Thompson seedless grapes just like darker raisins, but they are oven-dried or treated with sulfur dioxide to prevent darkening. They are sometimes called sultanas, the name they go by in England. Because grapes are some of the highest-pesticide-residue fruits, it is a good idea to select organic raisins.

Per Serving: Calories: 244; Protein: 4g; Cholesterol: 0mg; Sodium: 184mg; Total Carbohydrates: 54g; Fiber: 2g; Total Fat: 2g; Saturated Fat: 0g

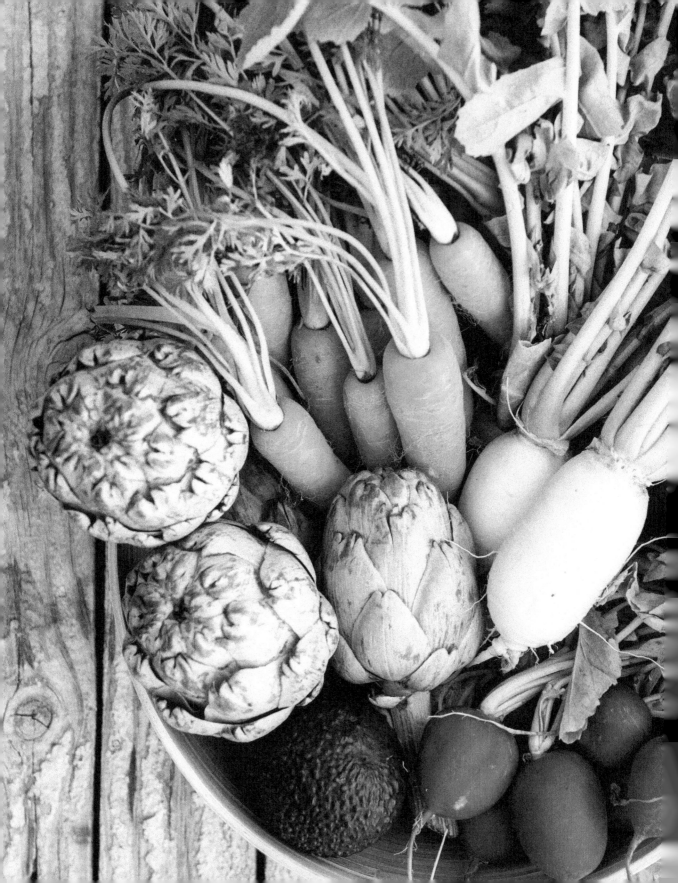

The Dirty Dozen and the Clean Fifteen

A nonprofit and environmental watchdog organization called the Environmental Working Group (EWG) looks at data supplied by the US Department of Agriculture (USDA) and the Food and Drug Administration (FDA) about pesticide residues. Each year it compiles a list of the lowest and highest pesticide loads found in commercial crops. You can use these lists to decide which fruits and vegetables to buy organic to minimize your exposure to pesticides and which produce is considered safe enough to buy conventionally. This does not mean they are pesticide-free, though, so wash these fruits and vegetables thoroughly.

These lists change every year, so make sure you look up the most recent one before you fill your shopping cart. You'll find the most recent lists as well as a guide to pesticides in produce at EWG.org/FoodNews.

THE DIRTY DOZEN

- » Apples
- » Celery
- » Cherry tomatoes
- » Cucumbers
- » Grapes
- » Nectarines (imported)
- » Peaches
- » Potatoes
- » Snap peas (imported)
- » Spinach
- » Strawberries
- » Sweet bell peppers

Kale/Collard greens & Hot peppers*

THE CLEAN FIFTEEN

- » Asparagus
- » Avocados
- » Cabbage
- » Cantaloupes (domestic)
- » Cauliflower
- » Eggplants
- » Grapefruits
- » Kiwis
- » Mangoes
- » Onions
- » Papayas
- » Pineapples
- » Sweet corn
- » Sweet peas (frozen)
- » Sweet potatoes

*In addition to the Dirty Dozen, the EWG added two produce items contaminated with highly toxic organophosphate insecticides.

Measurement Conversions

Volume Equivalents (Dry)

US STANDARD	METRIC (APPROXIMATE)
⅛ teaspoon	0.5 mL
¼ teaspoon	1 mL
½ teaspoon	2 mL
¾ teaspoon	4 mL
1 teaspoon	5 mL
1 tablespoon	15 mL
¼ cup	59 mL
⅓ cup	79 mL
½ cup	118 mL
⅔ cup	156 mL
¾ cup	177 mL
1 cup	235 mL
2 cups or 1 pint	475 mL
3 cups	700 mL
4 cups or 1 quart	1 L
½ gallon	2 L
1 gallon	4 L

Volume Equivalents (Liquid)

US STANDARD	US STANDARD (OUNCES)	METRIC (APPROXIMATE)
2 tablespoons	1 fl. oz.	30 mL
¼ cup	2 fl. oz.	60 mL
½ cup	4 fl. oz.	120 mL
1 cup	8 fl. oz.	240 mL
1½ cups	12 fl. oz.	355 mL
2 cups or 1 pint	16 fl. oz.	475 mL
4 cups or 1 quart	32 fl. oz.	1 L
1 gallon	128 fl. oz.	4 L

Oven Temperatures

FAHRENHEIT (F)	CELSIUS (C) (APPROXIMATE)
250°F	120°C
300°F	150°C
325°F	165°C
350°F	180°C
375°F	190°C
400°F	200°C
425°F	220°C
450°F	230°C

Resources

Explore the resources provided here for more information on the microbiome.

GENERAL INFORMATION

» **American Gastroenterological Association (AGA) Center for Gut Microbiome Research and Education**
www.gastro.org/about/initiatives/aga-center-for-gut-microbiome-research-education

» **American Microbiome Institute, nonprofit organization, established in 2013, dedicated to advancing microbiome science and education**
MicrobiomeInstitute.org

» **The Clinical Guide to Probiotic Products Available in the United States**
USProbioticGuide.com

» **The Clinial Guide to Probiotic Supplements Available in Canada**
ProbioticChart.ca

» **Gut Microbiota for Health**
GutMicrobiotaForHealth.com

» **The International Scientific Association for Probiotics and Prebiotics**
ISAPPscience.org

MICROBIOME BOOKS

Blaser, Martin J. *Missing Microbes: How the Overuse of Antibiotics Is Fueling Our Modern Plagues* New York: Henry Holt and Company, 2014.

Mullin, Gerard E. *The Gut Balance Revolution: Boost Your Metabolism, Restore Your Inner Ecology, and Lose the Weight for Good!*. New York: Rodale Books, 2015.

Sonnenburg, Justin, and Elizabeth Sonnenburg. *The Good Gut: Taking Control of Your Weight, Your Mood, and Your Long-Term Health.* New York: Penguin Books, 2016.

Yong, Ed. *I Contain Multitudes: The Microbes Within Us and a Grander View of Life.* New York: Ecco, 2016.

MICROBIOME RESEARCH AND TESTING

» **uBiome: Personalized microbiome screening and sequencing tests**
uBiome.com

» **Day Two: To sequence your microbiome so that you can get a diet that is personalized to predict blood sugar responses to thousands of different foods**
DayTwo.com

» **Openbiome: A nonprofit stool bank, expanding safe access to fecal transplants and catalyzing research into the human microbiome**
OpenBiome.org

FERMENTATION SUPPLIES AND RESOURCES

Katz, Sandor Ellix. *The Art of Fermentation: An In-Depth Exploration of Essential Concepts and Processes from around the World*. Chelsea Green Publishing, 2012.

» **Cultures for Health: To purchase starters to make your own kombucha, yogurt, sourdough, and more**
CulturesForHealth.com

References

Albenberg, Lindsey G., and Gary D. Wu. "Diet and the Intestinal Microbiome: Associations, Functions, and Implications for Health and Disease." *Gastroenterology* 146, no. 6 (2014): 1564–72. doi:10.1053/j.gastro.2014.01.058.

Campbell, Kristina. *The Well-Fed Microbiome Cookbook*. Berkeley: Rockridge Press, 2016.

Chassaing, Benoit, Omry Koren, Julia K. Goodrich, Angela C. Poole, Shanthi Srinivasan, Ruth E. Ley, and Andrew T. Gewirtz. "Dietary Emulsifiers Impact the Mouse Gut Microbiota Promoting Colitis and Metabolic Syndrome." *Nature* 519, no. 7541 (2015): 92–96. doi:10.1038/nature14232.

David, Lawrence A., Corinne F. Maurice, Rachel N. Carmody, David B. Gootenberg, Julie E. Button, Benjamin E. Wolfe, Alisha V. Ling, et al. "Diet Rapidly and Reproducibly Alters the Human Gut Microbiome." *Nature* 505, no. 7484 (2014): 559–63. doi:10.1038/nature12820.

FairShare CSA Coalition. *From Asparagus to Zucchini*. Madison: Madison Area Community Supported Agriculture Coalition, 2004.

Feltman, Rachel. "The Gut's Microbiome Changes Rapidly with Diet." *Scientific American*. December 13, 2013. www.scientificamerican.com/article/the-guts-microbiome-changes-diet/.

Glenn, G. R., and M. B. Roberfroid. "Dietary Modulation of the Human Colonic Microbiota: Introducing the Concept of Prebiotics." *Journal of Nutrition* 125 (1995): 1401–12. www.ncbi.nlm.nih.gov/pubmed/7782892.

Green, Katherine. *Home Fermentation: A Starter Guide*. Berkeley: Sonoma Press, 2015.

Kellman, Raphael. *The Microbiome Diet: The Scientifically Proven Way to Restore Your Gut Health and Achieve Permanent Weight Loss*. Boston: Da Capo Press, 2014.

Koeth, Robert A., Zeneng Wang, Bruce S. Levison, Jennifer A. Buffa, Elin Org, Brendan T. Sheehy, Earl B. Britt, et al. "Intestinal Microbiota Metabolism of L-Carnitine, a Nutrient in Red Meat, Promotes Atherosclerosis." *Nature Medicine* 19, no. 5 (2013): 576–85. doi:10.1038/nm.3145.

Ley, Ruth E., Peter J. Turnbaugh, Samuel Klein, and Jeffrey I. Gordon. "Microbial Ecology: Human Gut Microbes Associated with Obesity." *Nature* 444, no. 7122 (2006): 1022–23. doi:10.1038/4441022a.

Mullin, Gerard E. *The Gut Balance Revolution: Boost Your Metabolism, Restore Your Inner Ecology, and Lose the Weight for Good!* New York: Rodale Books, 2015.

Ridaura, Vanessa K., Jeremiah J. Faith, Federico E. Rey, Jiye Cheng, Alexis E. Duncan, Andrew L. Kau, Nicholas W. Griffin, et al. "Gut Microbiota from Twins Discordant for Obesity Modulate Metabolism in Mice." *Science* 341, no. 6150 (2013): 1241214. doi:10.1126/science.1241214.

Schrezenmeir, Jürgen, and Michael de Vrese. "Probiotics, Prebiotics, and Synbiotics—Approaching a Definition." *The American Journal of Clinical Nutrition* 73, no. 2 (2001): 361s–64s.

Sonnenburg, Justin, and Erica Sonnenburg. *The Good Gut: Taking Control of Your Weight, Your Mood, and Your Long-Term Health.* New York: Penguin Books, 2015.

Tobacman, Joanne K. "Review of Harmful Gastrointestinal Effects of Carrageenan in Animal Experiments." *Environmental Health Perspectives* 109, no. 10 (2001): 983.

Wu, Gary D., Jun Chen, Christian Hoffmann, Kyle Bittinger, Ying-Yu Chen, Sue A. Keilbaugh, Meenakshi Bewtra, et al. "Linking Long-Term Dietary Patterns with Gut Microbial Enterotypes." *Science* 334, no. 6052 (2011): 105–08. doi:10.1126/science.1208344.

Wood, Rebecca. *The New Whole Foods Encyclopedia: A Comprehensive Resource for Healthy Eating.* New York: Penguin Books, 2010.

Ziedrich, Linda. *The Joy of Pickling: 250 Flavor-Packed Recipes for Vegetables and More from Garden or Market.* New York: Harvard Common Press, 1998.

Recipe Index

Index

Acknowledgments

I want to thank Talia Platz, Katherine Green, Andrew Yackira, and the entire Rockridge team for their work putting together this book.

It is a very exciting time to be working in the microbiome space—when discoveries are being made on a daily basis. I feel very fortunate to be able to bring this science to a wider audience. I would also like to recognize the professionals who have come before me in writing about the microbiome. In particular Dr. Gerard Mullin who is a wonderful mentor to me and has been from day one.

To my father, who loves reading medical journals, and my mother, who still clips out articles and mails them to me, thank you for always supporting me.

To my husband, Reid, who is always my first editor.

About the Author

DANIELLE CAPALINO, MSPH, RD, CDN runs a private practice in New York City where she provides nutrition-counseling services with a specialty in digestive health. She is a registered dietitian with degrees from the Johns Hopkins Bloomberg School of Public Health and MIT. Danielle is the author of *Healthy Gut, Flat Stomach* and has written several articles for *The Huffington Post* on issues regarding food and digestive issues. Learn more at DanielleCapalino.com.

CPSIA information can be obtained
at www.ICGtesting.com
Printed in the USA
BVOW11s0022230317

479109BV00001B/1/P